Inside the Insane

Erica Loberg

chipmunkapublishing
the mental health publisher

Erica Loberg

Published by
Chipmunkapublishing
PO Box 6872
Brentwood
Essex CM13 1ZT
United Kingdom

http://www.chipmunkapublishing.com

Edited by Aleks Lech

Chipmunkapublishing gratefully acknowledge the support of Arts Council England.

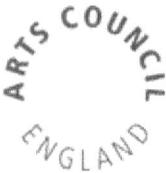

Author Biography

Erica Loberg was born in 1977 and raised in Westwood, California. She received her Bachelor's degree in English from Columbia University.

In 2005, Erica was diagnosed with Chronic Hypomania. She has worked with the mentally ill in Los Angeles County hospitals for over two years. This experience inspired her to write *Inside the Insane*. Currently, Erica lives in downtown Los Angeles.

Inside the Insane is dedicated to Erica's mother Mary Elizabeth Loberg.

Erica Loberg

July 2, 2008 – THE FIRST DAY

It was like going through an earthquake all fucking day. I walked into the dungeon with locked doors every few feet and that hospital smell that seeps into your fingers and nests in your fingernails and no matter how much you try, you can't shake the thought that you are going to have to get used to that smell. That greasy, sick, been-in-bed-way-too-long-with-no-soap stench that made my empty stomach find itself vomit to suppress the look of white fear on my shock-waved face.

I have to tell you I didn't expect to be so close to crazy, and I mean crazy unlike any crazy I've ever slipped as a normal word that people use without any consideration to the real meaning until it's walking down a hall with slice marks on its neck while you kneel down to speak to a patient that tried to kill her mother and needs to hear her options for her next move out of the hospital. It's something like that.

I think my white face turned to shaking hands when I walked by a woman in a room in solitary confinement standing watching a wall, then moments later I heard a bang and a raucous explosion as she tore off her clothes and smeared her feces on the walls.

I started to pray to my grandfather's spirit. He used to work in a hospital delivering babies and my mom said she never saw him because he worked so hard. I figured a hospital smell must have felt like home to him, so I called out to him for the ability to smell the tiles and walk by bodies with uniforms and an elevator that overruns itself then stops with a drop, so much that anyone on the brink of I may just barf right about now would. And I felt the yearning to feel something calming enough to walk forward and swallow fresh without a cold palm or deep bowel eruption. Calling on a dead one that you never knew to love, but do regardless, does the job. He was something there for me to focus on and it made me breathe, which was the hardest out of all the hard things to do that first day. Breathing was Mount Sinai.

The day started out peacefully. I sat in a meeting with a table of doctors, interns, psychiatrists and social workers. We went through all fourteen patients and spoke about their current mental status. The attendant sat at the head of the squad when the alarm went off like a fire bell.

"Erica, did you lean on the alarm?" He smiled and I sat up real straight without realizing he was kidding. Turns out it wasn't me. There was an episode in the hallway that required the alarm for assistance. It was called a Code Blue. A Code Blue was called if a patient had an outburst that required a team of people to come as fast as possible to assist in wrestling the patient to the ground, injecting him with tranquilizing meds, then tying him or her down in restraints on all four corners of the bed. Sometimes I would hear it in the lobby waiting for the elevator to take me to the 9th floor.

"Code Blue, 9th Floor. Code Blue, 9th Floor." It was announced by a recording of a calm woman with an easygoing inflection in her voice. It was used for severe situations on the ward. It was my first day and the code was called. That bell must have been used two weeks ago when a nurse was pulled into a room by a 300-pound patient and thrown on the floor to be raped, and barely escaped thanks to that alarm. She's now at home resting for a few weeks because she's dealing with shock. That's another type of earthquake.

Sometimes you're hardcore, you're outside of yourself, your brain, and your living known experience and then something happens. You are driving down the fast lane on the freeway and a belt of manic hyper voice releases from your lips and you grab the wheel and drive hard in your crazy moment that is, or was, "total control," to oh whoa, I'm on the side of the peel that is biting and ugly and time runs wild and you're somewhere else but still somewhere so it's not a problem.

Is that mania?

Is that mania?

Is that what constitutes mania?

Because since I've been here I've seen people outside of their orbit or any solar system I ever dreamed existed.

And then I look down at the sheet of current patients and it says BAD. Which is code for Bipolar, and I wonder, did I make a mistake? Am I bipolar or just an asshole making excuses for self medicating habits like joints and wine? I know that when I first had medication I felt excessive energy cease and it felt like, for the first time, I could drive without severe underlying urgency, or loss of breath inside my seams. But that's not worthy of institutionalization. I have not met these "bipolar" people, yet. And I wonder if they are bipolar one or two and for some reason there is no bipolar two recognized on the ward, or at least among the patients I'm with, for now.

Definition of Bipolar I
Manic-depression: Alternating moods of abnormal highs (mania) and lows (depression.) Called bipolar disease because of the swings between these opposing poles in mood. A type of depressive disease. Not nearly as prevalent as other forms of depressive disorders. Sometimes the mood switches are dramatic and rapid, but most often they are gradual. Mania often affects thinking, judgment, and social behavior in ways that cause serious problems and embarrassment. For example, unwise business or financial decisions may be made when an individual is in a manic phase. Bipolar disorder is often a chronic recurring condition.

Definition of Bipolar II
Hypomania: A condition similar to mania but less severe. The symptoms are similar with elevated mood, increased activity, decreased need for sleep, grandiosity, racing thoughts, and the like. However, hypomanic episodes differ in that they do not cause significant distress or impair one's work, family, or social life in an obvious way while manic episodes do. Hypomanic people tend to be unusually cheerful, have more than ample energy, and need little sleep. Hypomania is a pleasurable state. It may confer a heightened sense of creativity and power. However, hypomania can subtly impair a person's judgment. Too much confidence can conceal the consequences of decisions. Hypomania can be difficult to diagnose because it may masquerade as mere happiness. It is important to diagnose hypomania because, as an expression of bipolar disorder it can cycle into depression and carry an increased risk of suicide.

Manic depression and bipolar disorder are the same thing. I was diagnosed with Bipolar II about five years ago. Being in a bipolar mindset is completely different from another strain of thought but I am not like these people. I started to think that I shouldn't be medicated and just deal, because these patients were incarcerated. So what if I never slept much and talked like a fire hose. I'm beginning to rethink my own mental issues, which I can no longer call a disorder or disease, because it's not. I might just be someone just like everyone else that has been leaning on my disease to explain so much when really, I am a bitch complaining about a thing that is nothing. It's not even a thing. It's a small hypomanic disorder, totally far from a bipolar condition. Chronic hypomania is "my condition". Then I look at the medical sheets and see the same drugs that I have tampered with over the past five years and wonder, am I not as chronic manic as I thought or believed I had to deal with all these years? Do I really need medication?

But...despite my current rethinking of my own behavior, I remember the first time I took medication I woke up not exhausted. I actually woke up not wanting to kill myself with unbridled tiredness. That may be the most prevalent sign of my rehabilitation. I could wake up awake, and not so deeply exhausted that I couldn't deal. I had endured a whole life of waking up wanting to die from no solid sleep and didn't know any better. I thought everyone woke up with a body and mind that was forced to rise from the sheets with fog. When I was a baby my mom said I didn't sleep. I would just sit in my crib waiting for the rest of the world to wake up. When I was an adolescent I would anxiously stare in fear at the clock, knowing that I hadn't fallen asleep yet, and it was 4 am which meant I had to get up in three hours (while my sister slept calmly beside me) and know that I would finally find sleep around 5 am and would be hit with a ready to die anger that would result in me wanting to kill someone when I had to get up to do my hair. Everyone knew in my family to let me be in the morning and not speak a word to me. They chalked it up to me not being a morning person. I thought I was not a morning person my whole life till I realized it wasn't that I wasn't a morning person, I was a normal hypomanic person. It was only years later when I had a first break and went into treatment that my mom told me she always knew something was off. Her mother was bipolar so the symptoms were already there. But in that generation there wasn't a word for it. In an affluent American family, manic depression stayed inside the house.

When I went home I took a shower, got out, and took another one. I poured a wide glass of wine, sat on my balcony and started to write. *Inside the Insane.*

July 3, 2008 – NATURE VERSUS NURTURE

Is it crazy or nature working with nurture? Maybe it's a dangerous mix of coming out of the wound with a mental disease and then having witchcraft parents sexually abuse you and so you're left with anal sex with your sister, and a web for a wrist of white lines to remind you that at 20, you did that to yourself.
"I want to go and have a life. I want a job." He sat at the edge of his bed, shoulders hunched like tired limbs after a race.
"Well we think it's better for you not to be in your old environment because it may not be healthy for you." Aka, you were in a gang and we don't want you to return to that place. And being in a gang-infested neighborhood never crossed his mind as a setback.
"I just need to be away from my family." And that is why family makes wounds that we eternally try to heal.
"OK. We can find a facility in Hawthorne for you."
"OK. Sounds good."
He nodded and his plastic rosary sat on a thread across his shirt next to his nightstand with two magazines. Then the nurse walked in with a panic looking face, looking for her pen that she misplaced.
"Did you see my green pen? I think I dropped it."
I thought to myself, why is she riffling through his closet and clothes and magazine drawer? It's an invasion of privacy. Only now do I stop and think that maybe a pen is hazardous. But I thought he was safe and ready to build a new life for himself, away from his white scars when she was adamant about finding her pen. I think she had a pen that she loved and lost it, not that she was afraid he had it and would hurt himself. He was on his way to making a life for himself and I am sure that will be the case. Mr. Senor Cross across his neck. It was the beginnings of a major theme that would run wild throughout the world of the mentally insane. I didn't realize it at the time, that religion was going to be a chronic condition for most of the patients on the ward. But thankfully Senor

Cross had a cross around his neck and not one that was swallowed like his roommate so Christ could be ingested, or stabbed in the stomach cause el Diablo was talking inside.

I walked into this hard walled world thinking it was something I never even gave a brief moment to think about, and now, it's beyond putting my socks on, or climbing a sand dune. It's something far known and beyond any trace of knowledge, but I am here, and have a special spirit or gift or ability or whatever you want to call it, to reach these people inside their eyes of no one knows me. I don't know myself, but that connection between not knowing yourself completely and having a person that doesn't either builds a thread of recognition of humanity; a brief moment of yes. Yes. I am not alone in my loneliness. That is what I have to offer and have for these souls that wander in the halls alone in their disheveled hair and shrunk shoulders among doctors and nurses and others that are just passersby. Inside there is something not them and them more than the others and that is what I will find and seek out to the best of my mind.

July 4, 2008 – WHAT'S THE DIFFERENCE

It's day three and the shock and fear factor is not physically showing itself in the draining of blood from my face, or slow backpedaling from the bed where a patient sat quiet and peaceful and heard about an outreach program while one of her roommates walked in circles rambling. And I am fascinated that after a couple of days I am already building a tolerance to... I still don't have a term for it, and wonder when or why this situation will become normal so that only those inside the ward know how to deal while the rest of the world sits at their desk in a cube eating Doritos and slamming soda. What's the difference? One is living on a psycho scale mixed with environmental toxins and find themselves in a square hall wandering around, and the guy in the square cube never knows chronic anything.

I'd rather not be in an institution, so help me God. But I'd also rather not be in a car alone with myself void of reasoning or thoughts for something better. People ride in their blue tooth vehicles spewing bullshit to dipshits on the phone and never stop to think if what they are doing really matters, if it's what they want to do or become or wake up to. They just do because it's all they know. Senor Cross never had a chance to know what he wanted. And now he has a chance to dream about what he wants, he doesn't know what that is, which puts him at a grand disadvantage, but at least he knows that he wants something, and is ready to make that something happen.

Later that day I ran into the guy the treatment team talked about in rounds earlier that morning. A patient tried to cut off his head cause he thought he gave Aids to his wife and unborn child because he had sex with two prostitutes. And THAT was the worst of his worries? Not the gash on his neck or the thoughts to kill himself out of harsh guilt over sex with two prostitutes. Why is it that men can sleep with a hundred prostitutes and never take a deep breath of reflection and another has two acts of sex and tries to decapitate himself?

Deep different convoluted systems of the brain I guess.

July 7, 2008 – WEEK TWO

It's week two and I haven't felt the need to puke, which is good. I carefully turned my head in the halls to see if anyone was in the secluded cell and, thank God, no one was.

"Where is that woman from last week?" I didn't think I would ever get that image from the first day out of my crippled brain. She was still around, somewhere. She had wild curly hair that sat on top of her head like giant cotton balls. When I first saw her she was in the seclusion room staring out the window. Then she would turn like a switch and bang on the walls screaming at the top of her wide lungs. The doctors and nurses were on top of it as they watched her agitated escalation on the monitor. Wrestle, inject, submit. They managed to keep her "down" enough to strap her to the bed in four point restraints. For now.
"ECT? I don't know. She's around." Nicaragua said it like it was Tuesday. She was training me for the job. Nicaragua was a five

foot nothing immigrant from Nicaragua whose family came to this country with nothing. She had a masters in social work and psychology and seemed to have seen it all.

"Oh." I really didn't want to know if ECT was "around" so was a bit relieved.

"Nicaragua, can I go home now?" It was the same guy from last week with the same shirt and the same tormented face with the same line.

"I put the paperwork in." Nicaragua said as she opened the door to the offices and closed him off.

"Here is your desk." She pointed to a nightstand with a foot of space for my notebook.

"Aquafina sits here." I was to share a hole with another social worker.

"She's kinda weird."

"Great." I found out later she was a little off. She worked hard through her offness so I did my best to deal the homo cards she seemed to give me. She was a lesbian who liked to drink my water when I wasn't around. Water that was in a closed Aquafina water bottle that sat in the corner of my nightstand desk. She also liked to doodle eyeballs in my notebook when she used my phone. She was watching me. Or maybe she just wanted me. But her bizarre behavior was the least of my problems.

Later that day Nicaragua and I did some paperwork and then Nicaragua went to visit a patient to see where she wanted to live in a voluntary facility.

"I can't be near my mother. I will try and kill her and go at her with a knife if I'm with her." You've got to love her honesty, and so she settled on a facility on the other side of her demon.

July 8, 2008 – HYPERSEXUALITY

Stamp. She was Asian. She was bipolar with a history of hypersexuality. She was also a prostitute, twenty-three years old, and was raped. She walked along the side of the hallway and Nicaragua approached her to talk to her about going to an Institution for the Mentally Ill, aka an IMI.

"Stamp, hi, I'm Nicaragua." She stopped suddenly.
"Hi."
"This is Erica."
"Hi, how are you?" I asked with a smile.

"I don't know, good, I don't know what to say." She was nervous to answer how are you because somewhere along the line it wasn't said right and now was on the bench of uncertainty. She stamped her right foot every few seconds and was my first Asian bipolar encounter, or Asian mental patient anything.

Hypersexuality took many forms and meanings on the unit. If you preferred to be naked and free ball it while strutting down the catwalk you were put on sexual precautions. Or if you were caught saying inappropriate sexual things, or reaching out and touching someone, also no good. To be honest, I was a little hazy on the matter cause I was clinically considered hypersexual and it took many forms in many different times in my life so I never had a clear understanding of the term.

July 10, 2008 – THE TIMES

"The Street. What are we going to do about The Street? Any ideas?" The doctor asked the treatment team.
"We can open the door and maybe he'll walk out." Rounds were on the lighter side today, yet, beneath that remark was the truth that after all the treatment in the world, sometimes you just don't know what to do with a patient. Oftentimes if you didn't know and there were no housing options they would be discharged "to self." In other words, to the street. But you wouldn't be caught dead saying such a thing, because you would be a dead career doctor. It was sacrilegious and a quick advertisement for the front page of the Los Angeles Times: Patient at Ocean View Medical Center was discharged to the street yesterday then found dead on the road by a bus stop after falling into a ditch when attempting to get help from a passerby. Or a patient can seem just fine and be discharged "to self" then found a week later dead on the cement in the Los Angeles River. The bridge is that high up but the water runs dry. It's interesting what doesn't make the Times. More importantly, what

gets covered up by a hospital. Over at Central Hospital a man hung himself around 10 pm with his torn shirt in the bathroom shower. His roommate found him hanging the next morning around 4 am. He thought he was having a regular one of his terrible hallucinations so went back to bed. Later around ten he woke up to the same dangling legs and called for help. When it hit the Times it was a big deal because people wondered what the 24 hour staff were doing all that time. They said they were dealing with another extreme patient situation that required lots of surveillance. As it turns out, the nursing staff had fallen asleep. But that didn't make the Times either.

July 11, 2008 – OCEAN VIEW MEDICAL CENTER

Ocean View Medical Center is considered the flagship of all county hospitals. It is a teaching hospital located in Southern California. There are two inpatient psych wards. The 2nd floor housed 15 patients and the 9th floor housed 30. Other than the number of patients the biggest difference between the two is the light. On the 9th floor there are windows facing south. There are no windows on the 2nd floor. Downstairs is known as the dungeon. Dark, dank, and a place where a sane person would plummet into depression in a mid-moment second. And a depressed person would fall deeper into the abyss of black hell.

The county employs me. I work for the Department of Crazy Health (DCH) as a county hospital liaison. The company I work for has contracts with mental institutions throughout Los Angeles County and works with the hospitals to find placement. As a hospital liaison I access patients on the ward that are then evaluated at my company and then referred to an institution. As a medical case worker it is my job to meet with the treatment team, and gather as much information about a patient as possible in order to present them to the gatekeepers so they can find the right place for them on the totem pole of incarceration. I was the one who met with the treatment team every morning to learn the latest of the latest craziness running down the halls then read the chart, wrote a synopsis, and then passed it over to the gatekeepers, the keepers of the locked gates who made the final decision on which gate a patient would enter. As a medical case worker it seemed like a go-between job, but so much seemed to appear between the cracks that could mean someone sits on a waiting list for a locked facility for months, or gets in tomorrow morning. It all seemed so arbitrary, yet, at the hospital level they have one purpose: get the patient stable enough so they can move them out, then pass them off to the next branch of the tree. I was the monkey swinging from branch to branch passing on information to the gatekeepers. Politically the hospital want their patients out, so the social worker's job is to facilitate that so oftentimes they tell me what they need to say and want me to hear to make sure this happens in a timely fashion so if a patient is acute they may spin a tiny lie and say they aren't. Yet, I know from the rounds that the doctor says something else. So what I choose to write for the gatekeepers to do their job and decide where a patient should go is based on summarizing input that swings through the trees, while information concerning the mental status of a patient falls here and there and the truth gets lost on the forest floor. I did my best to communicate the truth about a patient to the gatekeepers, but truth doesn't discharge patients fast. Truth would keep them in the ward long enough to stabilize them, which could take days, weeks, months. At 2400 dollars a bed a night, the county didn't have that kind of money for all the detergent needed to clean the sheets.

July 12, 2008 – HELP IS HERE AKA HIH

This morning I sat in the common room while Nicaragua spoke with a patient about going to an HIH. The Help is Here Program. HIH was a voluntary program for patients who needed assistance in the community once they were discharged. The program was new to me but it sounded like a good idea. A disheveled black man rolled himself into the room in a wheelchair. He had a dirty Afro, slouched shoulders, and a mean frown across his face.

"Hi." I was being friendly.

"Hi. I'm Pissed Off." I recalled the meeting earlier that day and how Pissed Off was a dead end case and wondered why.

"How are you?"

"I'm pissed. I had a clean white shirt in my locker to wear outside and they take it. These assholes hate me."

"I'm sure they don't hate you. They are trying to help you." I felt so stupid saying anything because if I were him, I could give a shit if anyone was trying to help me when I just wanted my shirt back. "No. They're assholes."

I let it go.

Later that night I emailed Carter. He was an old friend (lover, weakness, whatever you call that person who is in between a friend and a boyfriend and never seems to leave the heart.) Carter was someone who I've had a sordid relationship with, which is a pathetic use of the word sordid for the years of loose situations, and sent him some of my writings about my first day from *Inside the Insane*. He read my document titled *crazy* which described my first day in the ward. And he wrote back "Are you at a special treatment center?"

What the FUCK?!!!

Followed with, "Seriously dude, you good?"

Any normal person would think what they wrote was a bad email, and sent out the wrong message. No. Sorry. That would be a way too easy way to deal with the feelings I had of him thinking I was institutionalized for some reason which really shook me to the core. When a person you know forever and have a longstanding deeper relationship with, but apparently doesn't have one with you enough to know the dick shit difference, thinks you're insane, it's baffling. Am I in a treatment center...dude you good? If he really thought I was at a special place why would he not call or even worse say "DUDE YOU GOOD?" That doesn't even make sense after a lifelong term of fifteen years of a friendship with that something else you try to avoid always resting on the side. Or maybe it's more like sauce on a steak.

It gets beneath my skin. It scoops out my insides because Carter is someone I cared about. Someone who has known me, and has had privy to information about me, and my struggles or travels with my mind, and he automatically thinks I'm at a special treatment center. It is so fucked up that I wonder when it will stop being in the forefront of my lobe or even in my conscience. Forget about the subconscious, that's going to be screwed for a while, if not forever.

Who you are inside and what you show on the outside are two people, for everyone. Have you ever heard your voice on an answering machine and eeek when you hear it because it's not you. Just like seeing yourself on camera, or in a photo. Do I really look like that? But when someone else you know and have known for years sees you for someone you aren't, or even used to be, it's that much worse. Carter thought I was in a special treatment center and I was working at one pouring insight into that world which was beyond anything I ever saw or felt. When you are manic depressive and there are people in your inner circle that know and sometimes see your struggles, you are forever going to be *that* person. Not OK. Not normal.

Bottom line. I'm upset because I am at such a great place in my life and would never in any terrible nightmare be in a place to be in a special treatment center, yet, someone that I thought knew me assumes that. When I am misunderstood, it's misunderstanding, and never anything else. So do I shake it off and chop suey it up to he misread my diary entry, or does it read that I'm in a special place so he has to think that or does he assume that because that's what he thinks of me? I think that's what he thinks of me. Terrible as that is to write, or hear over and over again in my mind, it's the sad truth. I made the mistake somewhere along the way of disclosing my life of hypomania. It's worse than a birthmark because it's a birthmark on your brain. People don't see it but they know it's there. You make the mistake of telling even your closest friends that you're manic depressive and they never forget or neglect to ask you "How are you doing?" It's never a simple question like everyone else gets. I am doing great. Just like everyone else OK! And you realize that a birthmark on your brain is an advertisement for "Are you OK?" for the rest of your life.

So, the question that I wonder if I will have to ask myself for the rest of my God given life: Do I drop him? Do I drop those that don't understand otherness? When you're finally not another type and have people close to you sending emails like that, you have to wonder, does this person know me? Maybe I've invested too much in a friendship that never knew the bedrock or roots beneath the surface, and took everything at face value and made judgments based on that mere façade of being.

But you need friends. You need some people in your life to carry the burden of knowing that you have a mental illness, as sad and unfortunate as that is, especially for those tiny palm full that make a difference. Like my best friend from kindergarten. Sloan. Sloan defined the meaning of a best friend filled with only unconditional love. She was there regardless of any given situation. She was my home. But no matter who you are, things change when you have your first mental break, and everything changed when I had mine.

CHAPTER 2

JOURNAL ENTRY - THE BREAKTHROUGH MOMENT - 2005

I don't think there is ever one breakthrough moment. I do, however, think bits and bits of pieces, days, nights, weeks, months of living in hell do eventually catch up with you. For me, my moment wasn't planned. It was one of the strangest, greatest, monumental moments in my life that was really a collection of dark times I've had for years.

It all unfolded pretty fast. One day I was walking down the street and every step I took was a terrible feeling of being in my own skin. I walked by a display window and caught a glimpse of myself. It didn't look like me. My brain had finally detached from my body and was ruling it, making it hard to find a way for them to co-exist together. I started crying uncontrollably and could feel my skin crawling on top of my hot blood. My mind was a complete pulsating blur and it emotionally hurt outside, finally. I called Sloan in a state of heightened trauma and bled through the phone.

"I can't take it anymore."
"Where are you?" I could hear the panicked concern in her voice.
"I can't take it."
"Where are you? I'm coming to get you."
"No. I can't. I can't take it."
"Take what?"
"I can't live in my skin anymore. My brain has melted it."
"I am coming to get you, are you home?" And like a switch I turned.
"I'm fine. I'm OK. I have to go." And I hung up, never thinking how hard it must be for my friends. I was so blessed to have friends that held on, especially when I couldn't. I walked back home and decided somehow, some way, I was going to get help.

The next day I was at the gyno having my regular examination. I sat on the table, completely defeated, with that stupid piece of paper falling off my back as the doctor wrote in my file.

"I need help." It came out of the air. I didn't think it before it dropped out of my lungs. It simply released itself into the room, nor did I think it was me who said it when it hit the oxygen. I sat there for a millisecond and wondered where it came from. It must have been the defeated self finally giving up. I had reached that bottomless pit and somewhere deep inside me something had had enough. It was the hardest and easiest thing I ever said. My doctor turned around as if I just told him Jesus Saves and said, "OK." Just like that. OK. And that was that.

The next day I was in a therapist's office with a plant and a Kleenex box resting on a glass table beside me and a clock staring back at me across the room and a woman watching me as I started to speak. Fifteen minutes into my monologue she stopped me.

"I'm not going to be able to help you." I thought she was kidding.
"Ah, OK."
"You are going to have to see a psychiatrist." I'm not quite sure what I said that made her say that. Maybe it was how I said it. I guess I was more messed up than I realized.

The next day I was sitting in a psychiatrist's office and that was the beginning of my recovery. My long forever in my life recovery that would be the beginning of playing hopscotch with meds.

"Hi." He sat down, comfortable in his reclining leather chair.
"How are you today?"
"Fine." The obvious answer to someone who is not fine and knows it. We went through the last 28 years of my life. My extreme boredom that plagued my existence because my mind ran so fast that life couldn't keep up with it. My sleeping habits, my activities, my piano lessons, my gymnastics, my sailing lessons, my dance classes, my Columbia degree, my high honors in everything I did. Did, but not now. The upper class society I grew up in had turned into a torpedo with fire bleeding from my skull. I'm sitting here now with a phone mumbling in my brain and limbs straight across my chest and what is this and can you help me. After two hours of my life on the table he came out with it so simply.
"You're hypomanic. Bipolar II." He uncrossed his legs, stood up,

and walked back to the wall dividing the patient from the doctor, the desk, and squashed down comfortably into his leather chair.

It was hypomania. An extreme state of hyperness that rose above a regular person's steady Sunday while I'm on fire all day would sit there every second of my mind.

It was pure enlightenment fueled by unbridled energy that was ready to die. And would soon be regulated. It was time.

And now, I look back, and wished I had some giant red flag bursting out of every sidewalk I sped down, every pillow I couldn't fall asleep on, every door that I opened to a scary future existence. But I didn't. It was only later in life when I began to truly dive deep to finding answers did I discover the red flags. Red flags that in hindsight could have saved me from years of ignorance to the realities of mental illness. And I found it in the writers that also suffered from bipolar disorder.

"The First Day's Night Had Come"
By Emily Dickinson

And Something's odd — within —
That person that I was —
And this One — do not feel the same —
Could it be Madness — this?

"Melancholia"
By Charles Bukowksi

there is something wrong with me
besides
melancholia.

"Earth, My Likeness"
By Walt Whitman

…there is *something* fierce and terrible in me eligible
to burst forth,
I dare not tell it in words, not even in these songs.

I look back and wish I had the knowledge to know that there were other writers who were bipolar and they also did not have foreknowledge to explain what that "something" was that sat inside their brain and turned out their insides.

JOURNAL ENTRY - SUMMER - 1998

I am going through *something* strange right now in my life, and I wish I could pinpoint what exactly my problem is. Problem is not the correct word, but I am short of any other word.

JOURNAL ENTRY - BREAKDOWN MOMENT - 2005

It must have been the defeated self finally giving up. I had reached that bottomless pit and somewhere deep inside of me *something* had had enough.

Looking back, years of manic depression could have been sought out. That word *something* could have been one of my red flags.

CHAPTER 3

July 14, 2008 - INSTITUTION FOR THE MENTALLY ILL AKA IMI

It was a smelly field trip and like a racetrack for the mentally deranged. Around and around and around they would go, walking in a loop around the facility waiting for a cigarette break. Nicaragua was showing me around town to the four IMI's that were sprinkled throughout LA. I sat in on one of the treatment rounds which occurred every three months for the inmates. Makes Sense to Me. She had a nice long strand of pearls and serious issues about seeing the dentist.

"If it doesn't feel good, it ain't good." It made sense to me and was her reason for not wanting to have her teeth checked out. Then there was The Stalker. She was a quiet Asian woman with a pink floral top. She had a restraining order for stalking a guy she was determined to marry so she wasn't going anywhere anytime soon. Next was Pick any Number. Pick any Number was a black man with twisted dreads that shot out of his head like antennas. The psychologist went through the list of questions and the rest of the treatment team responded on a scale based on their own needs or experience with the individual: 1.) How is he physically? 2.) Intellectual function, 3.) Response to stress, 4.) Thought process, 5.) Social interest. I give him a 2..4..1..8..3. The numbers seemed to be tossed out into the air based on people's moods at the time. Those numbers determined whether or not the jailed could move onto another racetrack that may have some outdoor space to get some air between your fingers when you smoked your cigarette.

"Do you know the names of your meds?" Always a question that seemed unfair, because it's not like every time they are forced to pop a pill they can recall the name of it. And since the doctors changed the dosage and type of meds to put a patient on practically EVERY DAY, how are they supposed to know anything? I didn't even know the exact milligram count of my own meds, for Christ's sake.
"I don't know." Pick any Number was providing honest answers to

the panel of queries.

"You're taking ...." The doctor ripped off about eight or nine different meds.

"Do you like the food here?" The cooking department was eager to hear if their culinary skills were up to par. The chef wanted to know if his inflatable eggs and dried out burrito tossed back with an OJ the size of half a swig was up to the standards of his culinary education.

"No. The food's not that good."

"You are 6'0" so you should weigh about…"

"I was 6'9" when I came from prison." The cook ignored his response and continued.

"When you go to the canteen get something healthy."

"I only have a dollar." The table was ready to wrap up the update as Pick any Number continued.

"Right now I'm finding myself. I'm not getting any younger. I got kids you know. I have a rap label and the meds are messing with my thinking." OK, so he wasn't a rap artist and didn't have any kids but he wasn't getting any younger and the meds were messing with his thinking so..he wasn't totally off.

"OK, thanks, sounds to me like you need more time to get your head straight."

And he was out and the final contestant took a seat. The Vice President. She had a black shirt with shiny fluorescent indiscernible images sprinkled randomly across her chest.

"We see here that you have been taking a lot of Motrin."

"I have a dislocated shoulder."

"Then you will need to see a doctor."

"No doctor. I don't want any CAT scan on my shoulder."

"You can't keep taking Motrin without a doctor evaluation."

"We'll see. We'll see." She was adamant and there was no chance for her to bend. The cook stepped in.

"Do you like the food here?"

"Since I've been the vice president I think it's a lot better. I heard people say they want steak which doesn't make any sense because we have no knife. People here do not have their heads on right enough to discuss their opinions."

And so it goes. They'll see her in another three months. Maybe by then she'll be president of whatever club discusses the lack of steak and no knives.

July 16, 2008 – MORE IMI'S

I visited some more IMI's today. I supposed since my job entailed placing people in locked facilities it would be a good idea to check out more places. I'd rather be a dog in a pound sitting on death row than at an IMI. And I'd rather be acute on the catwalk inside a ward than live in a dingy doll's house establishment with the curtains laying low, and a line of airport chairs to sit on with him or her next to you, or do they have assigned seating at 2:45 in the afternoon when I happened to drop by and the patients are there doing nothing. In terribleness. Nothingness at least is nothing but terribleness is terrible. I found out later that no one working in the hospital had ever been to an IMI. Zero of the residents or doctors (who determine a patient's level of care) had any vague idea of the insides of these places. They sent people to a place they've never been. I didn't get it that they didn't get it. They never saw the guy sliding down a chair half dead and stuck in some type of purgatory mental coma. They were all locked and desolate and they reeeeked. They reeked like grim on top of grim toe jam. Patients did what most patients do all day. They slept in their beds or walked in circles like slow greyhounds in a race. A race to go nowhere.

July 20, 2008 – LEVELS OF DANTE'S HELL

The level of care for a patient was an upside down totem pole of recovery. You start on one level and if you do well you graduate to a lower level of care all the way down till you hit the ground floor and could walk away back out into the world. Maybe. That was the goal.

TOP

Top was just that. The top. It was a state hospital that took prisoners of the mind and warriors of the human condition and locked them inside a wired box. I never stepped foot inside so won't pretend to know the screams of agonies crippling the soul that mustard all over the place, but I knew that at some point I would come across patients from there, or going there, and that was that.

Erica Loberg

THE SUBACUTE FACILITIES – Sunny Side & Shoreline

I visited the subacute facilities today, which is a step below Top, and a higher level of care than the IMI's. It had its amenities like a pool and space to move your ankles when you sat on the airport chairs but it also had locked doors that were banged on when the cigarette break was two minutes late. I was not a smoker but I would definitely pick up the vice just to have something to look forward to. Sunny Side was spacious, clean, or cleaner than garbage, with colorful walls. And the wall on the outside that people could go awol over is easier than a kid trying to get over a shitty pool gate to go for a swim when he will most definitely drown. It was all ass backwards. If you were badly off and paced too much you got to be in a wing with lots of open space. Open space versus a hallway to walk down until you rounded a corner to the next one then were back at the beginning, and it had been twenty three times so far that hour.

Later that day we hit up Shoreline. Shoreline was for senior citizens. I wasn't quite sure what to make of the place. I still don't. Shoreline was far from peaceful. It was the equivalent of Sunny Side but for 58 plus year olds. When I visited I almost cried. It was break time and all the patients were outside on hot cement eating popsicles. Before I could take it all in I was stopped.
"You're an ugly bitch." She or he, I wasn't sure because the place had turned this patient into an it, approached me.
"Thank you." I ended up backing away and out to stop the strings of spit that hit my clothes and face. Shoreline was old sadness. A place to die after a slow death.

ENRICHED BOARD AND CARE

Again, sounds good. I like the word enriched. It sounds comfortable and soothing. Ah..no. An enriched board and care was one step below an IMI and one step above a regular board and care. They were an open setting so patients could come and go as they pleased. They had groups and access to medication and a bed in a room to share with a roommate that you may not like but had to deal with because this was not college where you could request a new roommate. They were dark, lonely, and filled with supreme boredom. Boredom that would hit the common room hard where one TV would be on at all times and a line of chairs would occupy a list of patients.

REGULAR BOARD AND CARE

Simply put: this was a place to lay your head. They were dark, dreary and filled with lost hope and never dreams. A board and care is one step above a shelter but at that point..what is the difference.

THE STREET, SHELTER, JAIL or HOME PLEASE BE SWEET HOME.

You can be discharged "to self" aka the street, or discharged to a shelter, or have to go back to jail. That is, if your parole officer can track you down, which may or may not happen if you played your fake social security card right and picked a random name to really throw them off. And, finally, home sweet home. Sweet if you were lucky to have that front door you grew up knowing open. But your family may be unlucky, and take back a patient that tried to drown the family dog after throwing a sibling out the window, however, that is a chance every family takes when they take home a family member hot off the catwalk.

July 22, 2008 – STRONG BODY STRONG MIND

Strong body strong mind. Several prison inmates work out. They don't let themselves go. In a mental jail, there were no gyms. No place to sweat or run in a straight line or work a pull down machine. I visited a schizophrenic kid today during his cigarette patio break and he was the only one doing push-ups. Then he took off his shoe to stand on so he could do calf lifts. His ten-minute break was ten minutes to do a push-up. Strong body strong mind. Without a routine work out schedule and simple access to a treadmill or stationary bike, how are you supposed to beat the battle within the mind? The body and the mind never divorce but somehow the system lacks the realization that working out is almost just as crucial as popping a pill.

"Have you been working out?" He sat in his usual chair in his usual stance with my file placed casually across his legs and his chair tilted back a bit, just to make sure no one was looking. Dr. Sampson. He was my psychiatrist.

"Yeah."

"How often?"

"Ah..three four times a week. I run."

"So last time we spoke you had starting working at Ocean View Medical Center. How's it going?" He made a note in his folder of my life.

"Good." I had been out of work for a long time. Months had turned to over a year that plummeted me into a depression of unknown strength. I was so thankful to have a job now that I knew the days of days of what am I going to do were finally behind me.

"Ocean is an interesting place." At least my psychiatrist knew something about what I faced every day.

"Yeah, it's pretty crazy. I'm wondering if I need to take so much dosage of meds." He scratched something else in my file.

"You seem to be doing very well on your meds."

"Yeah, I guess so. I just see so much over-medication and patients that are far worse than me. I just wonder if I need as much."

"We can lower your meds and see how it goes."

"OK." We lowered my mood stabilizer by 100 milligrams, making my daily intake 200 in the morning and 200 at night.

"Have you thought about therapy?" I was waiting for the question that he managed to ask me every goddamn time. Usually it was followed by a lecture on how it was something I desperately needed. Therapy was a luxury that I couldn't afford. It was a dead end and I hoped one day the issue would stop walking across the carpet.

"When do I have to see you again?"

"How about six weeks?" He flipped his calendar and penciled me in and handed me a card with the date and time neatly printed on it. I knew six weeks from now I'd forget the date and the time of my appointment and have to call him for it.

"Sorry I have called you the past few times because I forgot my appointment."

"It's OK. Maybe you subconsciously don't want to come see me so forget."

"Yeah, maybe you're right." It's not that I didn't like to see him, I liked Samps, it was just burdensome and nothing has really changed in my life or behavior since I started working again and, more importantly, finally, my fucking God finally, the medication seemed to be right. At least for now. I walked out feeling good that I went and that it was over and that the next visit was set farther down the road than the last time. Maybe I was truly getting better. Thank you again God for finding me the right river to swim in. The meds were finally working, I think. You're never really sure though because once you find a medication better than the ten other ones you tried and drowned in, you stick to it, because you don't know what would happen if you jumped into another body of water. You could be faced with a tidal wave or caught in a dismal dead pond. And all the life below the surface you would have to live with. The depths of society are just as terrifying as the body of water you swim in. And so is the land that surrounds you. Later in life I found similar metaphors that strung through bipolar writers. Imagery to describe a mental state. Diction that caught a moment in time to describe that state. And my favorite, the only other bipolar II writer I knew as my own, was Samuel Taylor Coleridge.

"The Rime of the Ancient Mariner"
By Samuel Taylor Coleridge

Alone, alone, all, all alone,
Alone on a wide, wide sea!
And never a saint took pity on
My soul in agony

MOUNT EVEREST

Get up.
The faint buzz of foggy nothingness
Is me
A zombie that walks to her home
I watch an episode of Sex and the City

29

I've seen it…four
Teen times?
I don't want to die
But I can't get up from my chair to return the video
The bathroom is Mount Everest
So I hold my pee
As long as I can
My mind is crying and crying
I can't find the tears
Or wipe them away
They just fall down my body
And fill my soul
The sea of salt
Depression
I can swim
With waves,
I may drown.

CHAPTER 4

July 26, 2008 - CPA

CPA. She didn't want to go anywhere but home. She was a CPA who had a psychotic breakdown at 40 something and lost her job and lost her house and tried to stab her husband of 20 years in the chest with a kitchen knife. Not totally sure about the ocean of events and stages that hit the surface, but it seemed to happen fast. Now she was in a room sitting on the edge of her bed, still, sweet and alone.

"CPA?" Nicaragua softly opened the door like she always did after her respectful knock. Last week we entered another patient's room to discuss the latest on his discharge plan and he was wrapped around in a white sheet lying flat like a mummy in his bed.

"Hello? We can come back later." He raised his head.
"I'm OK."
"If you want some more time to sleep, I can come back." He melted back into his sheets and she walked down the hall, papers across her chest, ready for the next thing in her day. With CPA, things were different following the soft knock.
"Yes." CPA slowly turned her head and Nicaragua entered.
"I would like to talk to you about your discharge."
"What do you want?" She had little trust in anyone off the hall.
"I want to talk about some options of where you can go after here."
"I'm going home." She said it with her firm lips and straight strand of gray hair that she combed so long down the stems that it was firm and uncompromising.
"OK, well..." Nicaragua tried to move on with her options post hospital.
"I'm going home." After 20 years of marriage she had not been told that her husband didn't want to take her back. She had not been told that her options would be a board and care or a subacute or an IMI. All she knew was that her hair needed to be combed. Maybe her husband was stopping by that day for a visit.
"OK." It was not up to us to tell her the truth. That would come from a social worker's mouth some time soon. We retreated and walked away. We walked back to the office and Nicaragua picked

up the phone.

"Who are you calling?"

"Her HIH. Hopefully she hasn't left yet." Nicaragua left a long apologetic message to the HIH to let her know she didn't have to come that afternoon and there was a knock at the door. It was the HIH. She was a tiny Asian woman.

"Do you speak Cantonese?" Nicaragua inquired.

"Yes." After hearing Nicaragua tell her the low down on CPA not wanting to go anywhere cause she was "going home" she still wanted to speak with her. We all walked down the hall to find CPA. The HIH entered the common room where CPA sat in a chair at the head of a table staring blankly at the air in front of her. The HIH immediately started speaking in Cantonese and they communicated. They spoke for a good 20 minutes and she was still not going anywhere but home. But she had a conversation, a conversation for 20 minutes, and made it clear to me that speaking to patients in anything other than their native tongue was pointless. Yes, CPA knew how to speak English, but culture is not just a language.

July 29, 2008 - CATATONIC

"You're too red to work here." ECT (Electroconvulsive Shock Treatment) was warming up to me. She had called me a conceited bitch the day before. I found out she had previously had over a dozen electric shock therapy treatments AND she was open to doing ECT, so I felt a little better about the whole thing. Then along came another patient who was thrilled to be moving out of the hospital to Sunny Side, "Whooo, hooo!!" He scurried down the hallway with his arms jumping up and down in the air in pure delight. Have you seen the shit hole you are about to live in? I suppose it's better having a moment of fun before you enter hell and even better to enjoy the idea of moving on than being restrained against your will and moved to a place you didn't know. He ran by Catatonic. I found out about Catatonic earlier that day in rounds.

Catatonia is a syndrome of psychic and motor-disturbances. In the current Diagnostic and Statistical Manual of Mental Disorders published by the American Psychiatric Association (DSM-IV) it is not recognized as a separate disorder, but is associated with psychiatric conditions such as schizophrenia (catatonic type), bipolar disorder, post-traumatic stress disorder, depression and other mental disorders, as well as drug abuse and/or overdose.

In other words, we are not really sure what the heck it is. It was like another PDNOS (paranoid but not otherwise specified). Since the doctors weren't totally sure where it surfaced from, or where it fell on the desert of crazy, Catatonic was a case study for us to try and learn something. He was a new admission. The whole treatment team walked down the hall and Catatonic was standing still with one arm straight out in front of him and the other by his side. The doctor spoke first.

"Hi, Catatonic. Can we talk to you for a moment?" Nothing.

"This is our treatment team, and we would like to ask you a few questions." Nothing.

"Do you know why you are here?" He made an eating motion. He was fiercely skinny and hadn't had anything but an orange in the last two days. He also had long thick nails with a hint of puss like yellow snot, but that was the least of his worries.

"Can I move your arm?" The doctor moved his arm to the side and Catatonic left it there like a diving board.

"Can I touch your forehead?" Before the doctor could glean the surface of his skin, Catatonic was on the ground on all fours staring straight ahead like a dog staring at a rat he's about to pounce on.

"OK, well not now. We'll come back another time."

Later that day, I walked back to my office hole, and Catatonic's mother was standing in the hallway, staring in disbelief at Catatonic's strange positions. Her face was white and her mouth was agape like she was staring at a terrible thing. She was still. He was still, then he walked over to the wall and starting playing his imaginary piano on it.

"Come on Catatonic, don't you want to watch TV with your mother?" The nurses were trying to get him to spend some quality time with his mom in the common room, but he just stood there. Then he walked over to his bed and rested his board of a back down on the mattress. A nurse took the pillow out from under his head to try and get him up and his head didn't move. It stayed there floating in the air sideways like he was still resting on the pillow. He didn't like to be touched and his mother had not moved since she got there.

Her face was stuck in stone and her puffy cheeks were now gray. I walked away and went to my hole to do some paperwork. Later when I walked back down the hall, I saw him in a catcher's stance near the floor. His mom was still stone but her eyes were blood shot, as the tears seemed to rake her eyeballs and never seemed to stream down her face. Maybe if she blinked her tears would get a break and pour out of her eyes but they were still, stoned, in a state of utter fear, shock, and unknowing pain. This was her son. She was his mother. This was his mother. He was her son. And neither of them could say a thing, or move, or touch each other. Not that they didn't want to, but they were in such a state of mental pain that that was all they could do. Just stand there and stare straight ahead with a deep face of nothingness. Nothingness in front of something unknown. A person beneath the cloud.

August 9, 2008 – JERSEY BOY

Things are going well on the ward. People were pissed but able to deal with their situation, most of the time. We had a manic guy from Jersey in rounds who lost it.

"You can't fuckin' talk to me like that." His boiling days were over and the eruption was no longer secondary.

"OK, you are going to have to leave now." The doctor got up and so did Jersey. He walked straight toward the other end of the room and behind me.

"I'm not leaving unless everyone holds hands together and walks out together." I leaned forward, not sure if I should ostracize him more by standing up or melt under the table. Across the table I saw a discharge planner on the team. She stood up and peeled away from the shaky beats of his face that were on manic overload. I stayed seated because it all happened so fast that he was out sooner than I could contemplate anymore about getting up out of my chair and out of the way.

THE KING OF THE IDIOTS

He came from Jersey
To walk to the Coliseum
To watch some game.

It's not clear what game that was
To enter a runway
And take a plane
To the Trojans
But he did it.

And he happened to walk
On the yellow dividing line
On the street
On his way to oz
And was stopped by police.

He sat in our office
With nurses
Doctors
Social workers
And was not happy to be there.

"I invented Facebook."
He talked about his friends getting better looking
As they get older
And everyone else got uglier
And that he was the king of the idiots
And he didn't get along with the Princess of France
Also roaming the halls.

Then he jumped out of his chair
In a crazed skin jiggling
Frenzy
Forget the mania in his eyes
When your face shakes in something intense
A thought
Or physical impairment due to mental derangement
You're riding a tumbling wave
He demanded to leave only if everyone else held hands

And walked out together.
The league of the idiots.

Jersey boy wanted to see the Trojan stadium so hopped a plane across the country. The following week another patient decided he wanted to meet Paris Hilton, so jumped a plane from Vienna and landed in the States. Sometimes in a manic mind you just gotta do something and you really don't have a choice in the matter because once that manic idea bolts through your brain, it's over. The next thing you know your whole steady life comes to an end. Change is good though. Immediate change is even better. But when you don't think things through because your mind doesn't let you, you will be stuck on board your bolt of lighting and nothing else can be said. Returning to your life before is not an option. You're getting on that plane.

CHAPTER 5

JOURNAL ENTRY - FALL - 1997

My first attempt to change began in my junior year in college. I was walking to the gym for yet another day of volleyball practice. It was my ninth year of volleyball and it was no longer a sport to me. I was just going through the motions like a mime with skill. I decided to stop by the office to speak to my coach about something that bothered me about her coaching, and didn't expect to walk out of the gym and never return.

"Hey Lobe! I never see you in here." I hated her nickname for me but somehow dealt with it.
"I just wanted to drop by and talk to you about something."
"Okay."
"I don't think I can do this anymore. I don't feel like it anymore."
"You don't feel like what?" I stared at her perplexed face that squeezed out of her terrible hair cut, hair that looked like she was a blind bull dike, and knew she was not ready for my next statement.
"I don't feel like playing anymore."
"A lot of people go through times when they hate their sport. That's part of playing."
I wanted to reach across her desk and pop off her tiny head.
"Yeah well that feeling has gone on for way too long and I have decided today to do something about it." I sat across the table firmly believing in the truth that was easily pouring out of my mouth.
"So you are just going to quit?"
"Yes." Tears streamed down my face. I didn't feel an ounce of pity for deserting her, because I couldn't stand the bitch. My tears stemmed from my ability to finally free myself from the burden of holding onto a sport that had become dead in me. It was like letting go of a dead animal that you carried on your shoulder for years and years, just because you always have. I was crying out of pure joy, because saying those words ended the internal struggle.
"You are going to regret this." She challenged me with her stupidity, and I looked her straight in the eye and said, "I don't think

so." And walked out of her miserable hole of an office.

I continued to cry and tried to pull myself together as I exited the building. I walked up the stairs out onto campus, and felt the weight lifted off my shoulders at every step I took. I did it! I QUIT!!!!! And it felt great.

The next day I walked across campus and decided I wanted to leave. I wanted to go and begin the deconstruction of Erica Loberg. I knew I had to go to a foreign place, and I was going to find the antithesis of city life. I walked into the study abroad office and sat down in the traveler guide's chair.

"I want to go abroad next spring." Like leaving volleyball behind, this impulsive statement came out of my mouth with no hesitation.

"Okay, where would you like to go?"

"I don't know...England...Ireland...Scotland...Australia...Spain." She didn't seem interested in guiding me through the process of nailing down a place or two for me to consider.

"Here is a book that explains the different programs. Why don't you look through it, and come back tomorrow, and we can see what's a good fit."

"Great, thanks!"

I walked home and started to read the information. Every program had the same perfect picture juxtaposed to a neat little paragraph describing how this place is the best place in the world to study. I realized that I was going to blindly pick a place and just go, so I did; London, England.

"London. I want to go to London." I was back the next day in the same seat chatting with the same woman with a part perfectly measured down the side of her head.

"We typically discourage our students from attending school in London. It is a busy place and can be an adjustment." Was she crazy? I go to school in New York freaking city and she thought London would be an adjustment?

"They do speak English over there?" She was not amused.

"How about Bristol? We have a great relationship with them, and have had great feedback from past students." She sold me in a second without any further investigation of my choice. The reckless impulsive behavior was shooting out of my brain so fast that it appeared to have no second to take a breath and actually think about my decision.

"Okay, Bristol it is then."

I filled out the paperwork and was ready for my new life.

JOURNAL ENTRY – ENGLAND SEMESTER ABROAD - 1998

When I landed in England I expected a cultural shock. No such luck. It was a lot of tea drinkers, and drinkers in general. I got settled in my little single dorm room and began the life change. The goal was simple: to learn moderation. To find a way to quiet the ongoing internal madness that bled my mind and flushed my soul. I had to find a way to stop being so hardcore. My life was an extreme measure dipped in fire and I was determined to find a way to become something else. I soon discovered that unfortunately changing your environment doesn't change your mind. My racing mind was stuck living in an environment where everyone was so slow and stale that every day was another ostracizing pill. I was in a foreign land. I only had a bed and a desk in my room which was isolated in foggy bushes of bleak nothingness. I had to walk five miles to campus, and only had to take two classes, (but still got full credit at my university), which was a bad thing for me. I needed books to shove down my throat and feed the hungry baby bird crying in the back of my brain. My life quickly slowed down and became a bit boring. I had too much time on my hands and no one to entertain me. I would take long walks and run and pray that my surroundings would curb my internal combustion. My moods were both confused by wallowing in the dark depressed environment, and feeling like a caged animal with nowhere to go. I would often kick box in my room and blow air punches at the mirror as I watched myself in my desperate attempt to release my fierce energy. My attempt at a "life change" was not going well.

CHANGE

Change
It's not hard
It's impossible
Drops of habit fill the holes of the brain
Which are formed over the lifetime of your existence
So now what?
Throw yourself on the floor
Rip the drops out of the holes
Through your nose?

Change happens with
Desperation
To eliminate the abysses
From the past
Subconscious forces formed in
Kindergarten.

Embrace the
Desperate need to change
Make demons your friend.

Not a drastic explosion of your kitchen
Acting out and feeding the hole with cookies
Literally.

Desperation scares away
All your ability to change.

Everybody wants change
Thinks about it
Ongoing
Dreams of it
To a hallucinatory state.

CHAPTER 6

August 11, 2008 - SCIENTOLOGY

The Scientologist was white and had something to say about the fact that she didn't feel comfortable being one of the only white people on the ward. She didn't like black people. She didn't like much. She was a Scientologist. At least that's what she tried to be before they threw her out. It was not clear to me if she was poisoned by the craft of Scientology bullshit driven acid forming nitrates on the soul, or was lost and off to begin with. Well, it's certain that she was like that to begin with because we are not born ready for dubious times, but still. The doctor came into my office to inform me that...

"We don't treat Scientologists."

"Oh, OK."

"They don't believe in medication so there's no point." But so many people on the ward didn't believe they needed medication, versus being in denial and not wanting to admit they're harmful without them.

So if Scientologists reject people, and they end up on the ward, and the ward shuts their doors to them, where do they go?

August 12, 2008 – SAINT JOHN THE APOSTLE

Saint John the Apostle was a young black kid with a bible glued to his fingertips. He was dying to go home and was often found dialing his father at the nurse's station. He was dialing a father who didn't have any intention of taking him home or any intention of telling him. I stopped to talk with him from time to time only to find all that time dedicated to Jesus. Jesus the savior of all good things. Jesus was John's answer to everything. Like so many patients in this world, religion was the answer to all.

August 13, 2008 – SLEEP WALKER

Sleep Walker was a young girl with a bad meth history and a history of sleepwalking when she was a youngster. Her habit was enough to make her end up on the street running away from her family. She had a father who was accused by everyone but Sleep Walker of molesting her.

"He was my best friend, my idol." Tears welled up in her dark brown eyes. Who's to say what was the truth, or the non-truth? Or just bits and pieces of what matters to glean enough information to make a clear assessment on why she was here in the psychiatric crisis ward sleeping face down, with one leg up like it was sitting in a chair upside down.

I let Sleep Walker sleep and decided to come back later to check on her. I wandered back down the hall and ran into...

Nametag.

"You can call me Gelesco. That's what you can call me."
"Is that your name? Why did you change it?"
"They call me that, you can call me that."
"What about your real name? You don't like that name?" She thrust her hospital bracelet out onto the scene in front of my face enough to see it. It read Nametag.
"I go by Gelesco."
"OK. How are you doing?"
"Are you a doctor?"
"No. I'm a medical case worker." It was the first time my title was said across the smelly tiles, or anywhere else for that matter. But that's what my tag said. At least finally I knew that and could justify wearing my chain of keys to enter the dungeon of walls inside severely deranged species that walked in circles, not for fun, but because their feet had to.

September 5, 2008 – HANJH?

I tried to do an HIH referral today for Hanjh? something (I am not sure how to spell or, more importantly, pronounce his name which is a problem when you are trying to build a relationship with a patient so they will trust you enough to trust that I am trying to help them.) I sat down next to him and his head hung low. Low enough to have a strained neck muscle scream out to him at some point and hopefully allow himself to pull his head up and not necessarily turn his head to see me, but turn it enough not to be hung by tired old threads of neck support. He was 62. He wasn't interested in talking to me. I thought maybe I'd try later and made my way to the next referral waiting for me down the hall.

Sleeping Now Awake was asleep in her bed when the nurse knocked on the door and flicked on the lights. The other three beds of wrapped cotton were still, not fixed on anything. Sleeping Now Awake rolled over to my face and ran her fingers across her eyes of sleeping now awake and smiled. I gave her the pitch of how this was a buddy system that had a person at her beck and call and maybe they will accept her. She listened while I threw in some bits here and there about my own funny need to let another person pry a little on me. And she smiled and actually let out a laugh. A real laugh from inside her skull into the air. Afterwards, I read her chart and saw that she was threatening and lashed out at people and stood on building tops ready to fly and wondered what made her laugh so cleanly, so nicely, so wholesomely and not needing to laugh but laughing because she was prompted to. Hers was a calm laugh. A calm laugh on the trail of screaming, hurting, tossing and turning in the halls. A calm laugh with so little to allow it to release. And I was there to hear it.

Later that afternoon I wandered the halls and stopped outside the seclusion room where a nurse I called Betty Boop stood on seclusion watch duty. She had an array of shirts straight out of a Disney store. They had cartoons on them and were painted in bright colors all over the front and back. All the nurses seemed to sport attire out of a Disney store. I didn't know if it was their uniform or whether a high-end nurse decided to wear it one day as a joke and the rest followed. Nurses were a clique just like the doctors, the residents, and the social workers. It was a high school cafeteria and I was shuffled somewhere in the bean mix. Betty Boop stood at the door.
"I came up with a dance today." I was ready to give her a break from her latex gloves and the dark circles under her lids.
"You're a mess." I wasn't used to the black lingo yet so thought she

Erica Loberg

meant I was all over the place when really mess was a term for crazy. Not a word one wants to hear on the ward but I let it go every time it fell on my ears.

"It's called the strap down." I strutted out the dance and her laughter bent her down over her Betty Boop jersey causing those around her to follow. Everyone needs a heavy laugh that bends the bones inside the asylum. The cleaning piss off the floor guy rolled his cart by and she stopped him.

"You gotta see this." His face lit up ready for something. It wasn't anything crazy or grand but fun. Fun was good. And it was accepted as funny. I did the strap down and he belted out a happy grin across his second day shadow of a face.

September 6, 2008 – MUSIC TO SAVE THE SOUL

I think these people need some tunes. They need to hear the rhythms of music to feel themselves again. Music stirs up the soul. We need to get some boom boxes in here and headphones for them to listen to. Some headphones next to their still silent beds. With music their streams of consciousness of feeling the self through the music and the flow of the stream of notes working together that mimic the rhythms found within the brain, may just make them feel better. Get them a jukebox. Then they can dance. Something.

SOOTHING INTENSITY

Sometimes music makes you laugh
Sometimes music doesn't make you cry
Sometimes it bleeds at the surface
Of your fragile skin
When you need it most.
Soothing intensity
That's the best way to describe it.
Music
Music from minds of beats
Thrusting moments
As is music
Intense
And of the layer
Underneath the outside.

I thought of the hard times in my life that I engulfed myself with music, stripping myself down to generate it into my skull. And that importance was a need, a must. Give them some music please. Something to match their torpedoed souls.

BI-POLAR

Axel Rose sings November Rain
I wonder about my problems
And why it hits my chord deep inside.
Do people beat and dance to the music like we do?
The chemically deranged?
Would you trade it?
No. Not in the moment but over time
A day
Of course.
You never know when it becomes lethal
Or too sad and pathetic
Because it's you.
It's you at yourself.

Is it a coincidence that music matches the rhythms of a particular mind that resonates with another similar brain? Or communicate similar feelings? The actual blending of notes to make a song may knock at your internal chords as two like minds form a bridge in music. Music may be a tool that can release the beats burning inside the skull. Music may also help discover a mental illness, not just in the lyrics, but in the way the music interacts with the brain.

A couple of hypomanics in music include:
Radiohead front man Thom Yorke and
Syd Barrett of the band Pink Floyd.

Axel Rose is manic depressive.

September 10, 2008 - I'M HUNGRY

CORN BREAK ON FRIDAY

Cornbread on a Friday
With a skip and a jump
Down the corridor
When aching moans of agony
And unknown explanations
Of pain
Seared down the hallway
Even patients were not amused
Or OK with the screaming
Remarks boiling
Out
Of the seams
Of an autistic mentally retarded patient.

And I smiled as I cut up
The cornbread
Into square pieces
For some long term social workers
Who were perturbed
And said
In their time
They've never seen such a thing.

And life was solemn
Inside the walls.

"He hasn't had a stool since he has been here." His name was I'm
Hungry. He was an autistic, mentally retarded 23-year-old who also
suffered from a mental disease. Rounds were on a demoralizing
note since no one, not anyone, could provide any insight to figure
out what to do with the giant baby standing naked in the seclusion
room yelling "I'm hungry" every few hours. And he hadn't had a
shit? I didn't understand it. It had been more than days riding on
weeksss…!

"I'm hungry, I'm hungry, please leave my mind." I walked by a room down the hall and a patient was rolling around in her bed with her hands blocking her ears that hid behind her stringy hair and I didn't know if she knew there was a screaming baby down the hall, or thought it was a voice in her head. I think it was a fair and honest statement that she wanted the voice roaring on the ward to cease. It didn't bother me, yet. But I also didn't have a broken rib from I'm Hungry's outrageous attacks at the nurse's station, or no sleep from working outside a clock.

September 16, 2008 – THE MAGGOTS

Since Ocean is a teaching hospital, oftentimes the attending would bring in a new admission to interview so the residents could learn more about aspects of mental illness. Although I enjoyed the learning process, sometimes I felt like it was exploitative. A patient would have to sit there at the end of a long table of about 15 people and answer questions. Since they were new to the ward, they were acute, so didn't really know what was going on or how to handle the questions but they did it anyway. Sometimes after the interview the residents would make flippant comments about the patient and didn't seem to have any insight into their strife or sympathy for their place in this world. However, sometimes the interview was helpful.

Today we had an interview with Maggots. She had legs full of maggots eating away at her crocodile skin shins. Thankfully she was first brought to the ER where they pulled them out one by one. God knows how long they were festering inside her boil looking shins. By the time she got up to the psych ward she was not so full of answers.
"Do you know why you are here?" The doctor asked in his usual gentle tone. She didn't feel like answering and the doctor continued.
"I know that you were on the sixth floor and you were treated for your legs. Can I see them?" She lifted up her pant and her leg looked like a log stuffed into a shoe so tight that the circulation was cut off, leaving the timber bulging purple log beneath thick old dry scabby stale skin.
"Can I see the other leg?"

September 18, 2008 – RECREATIONAL THERAPY

The patients had recreational therapy twice a day. It was voluntary but something that was charted to show if the person was solitary or engaged with peers. The activities were usually drawing or an art project with glue and shiny beads or a crossword puzzle. All the activities available during group time were geared toward a child. If you walked into a room during group time, you would see a table found in a kindergarten classroom and quiet students working on their project. If you were disruptive, just like in pre-school, you were asked to leave. Nail Polish had been through several foster homes before she found her biological parents at 20 years old. She told her mom she was going to kill her father when he got home and now she sat next to me (while we painted our nails during recreational therapy) and she was worried about paying 300 dollars for a home that would take her money, like the last one that had kicked her out onto the street.

"I can't be homeless again." I knew her parents would not take her back and so did she, finally. And I assured her there would be people to care for her and give her a home and she said OK with assurance and unknown okayness. Then I watched as she put a coin into the pay phone that the patients pay for with money from who knows where, and spoke to her dad. She cried that she didn't have a place to go, and tears streamed down her soft white skin outside her black dyed hair and I told her I'd take care of it. She was adamant about knowing she would have a single room. Her privacy. And I told her it would be like a dorm with a roommate. She rocked back and forth on the edge of her chair swinging in the information and said OK, OK. But I knew it was not OK. None of this was OK because she was here. She was inside the ward and had no idea what was coming after, where she would go, or how she would get money to pay for it.

"Can they give me SSI? I don't want to end up back on the streets." I had no concrete answers because I saw people let out on the street and thought somehow this wouldn't happen to such a solid soul trampled by schizophrenia, and even though her family was a phone call way, she was a person slung into the hospital to fend for herself.

It seemed so hard and soft at the same time.

September 19, 2008 – RELIGION ON CRACK FOUR THOUSAND AND...

Saint John the Apostle was discharged today and thankfully the bible left the armpit of his arm. The pious demons of the world are killing the sanity of the soul. Religion was a lifetime curse for most of the people on the ward. It ruled them to the point of insanity.

September 20, 2008 – IT WAS THAT BAD

It Was That Bad, a schizophrenic artist in seclusion, spent two hours on the ward screeching, "Let me out!!!" She was smart, and artistically accomplished, and stuck in a room yelling at the seams of her tongue and all we could do was observe her on the screen at the nurses' station because the window into her room was steamy, like a window looking into a sauna with finger prints on the fog of the glass. It was sad. Medication was not working and the pain was excruciating. The constant random yelling echoed the "I'm hungry" autistic mentally retarded giant child stuck in a baby's brain on the other ward. Repeated screaming bursting from lungs for hours off and on for days on end can never be expressed in any written words. You simply had to hear the drilling noise ricochet off the walls inside to begin to find an ounce of knowing. I'll never know and I was there. It was that bad.

September 21, 2008 - PINKY

PINKY

Pinky
Pinky had a hole in her foot
And was afraid that she didn't know it was there
And that she had to take care of herself
And she knew that

Now
In the walls of the ward of crazy
"I have to take care of myself."
And she would. Physically
Maybe
And let's hope mentally.

Society thinks mental illness is not a physical thing since it's not visible on the outside of the body. It's not a broken arm. But it is a broken mind. And it's the eyes that tell the story and connect the body to the mind. If you look straight into the eyes of someone suffering from a mental illness, you'll see something, you'll see it locked inside.

TO THE INSIDE

Depression lodges itself in the lids
Mania stirs itself in the eye
And eyes tell a story
A physical
Gateway
To the inside.

September 24, 2008 – FUSS BALL WITH A PAPER BALL

I had to make an effort now, more so than before, to spend time with the patients. I walked into the rec room and Fuss Ball was sitting there hunched over, like always.

"You want to play fuss ball?" He nodded and we walked over to the table and we both looked for the ball. We searched around the table, inside and out, and finally he pointed at a crumbled up ball of brown paper.

"I guess this is the ball." I smiled ready to play with a brown paper bag. We tried to play but it was too small to be hit when it was in between the red and white men. So I made another one out of the few pieces of newspaper that sat beside the airport chairs in a line and balled it up bigger than the brown ball and placed it on the table. We played. It worked in its pathetic paper way, slow, but a new game. It was fuss ball in slow motion. A real ball might get coughed in someone's suicidal throat or thrust up some hypersexual ass. You never know.

After the game, which started as best out of three then turned into best out of five, he asked me for a hug. I paused, not sure if that was in my boundaries. Was it wrong? Was it bad to touch a patient in an embrace? My hesitation turned to an OK and I did a pathetic bend waist through the chest hug that was returned, enough for him.

I wonder how much lack of physical contact ruined people. As bodies living within the mind within the ebb and flow and give and take and up and down of the being, it's the body and the mind that drives the being. Do we ever stop and realize they are one and the same? They are just as needful as lemonade needs sugar.

I hugged him and felt bad after that he had to ask, and I had to think about it, and it was more important than talking and evaluating the outside external experience of the world that was not touched with human warmth. To sleep in a bed alone all day in the dark with the covers over your head and slow walking alone up and down the catwalk, where is the human touch? Where is the other half of the self?

October 7, 2008 - CRITTERS

First there were maggots and then there were wigs with lice flying through the air onto the floor all over the place. I'm not sure which situation was worse but they were both little white critters so you be the judge. I continued to be surprised about the filthy realities of the human condition. It almost bothered me more than religion. Religion was also taking its toll.

October 8, 2008 – THE EXORCISM

We had an exorcism today with a priest and holy water and everything. Again, religion seemed to be doing much more bad than good, at least in the minds of those not living clearly. So thus far, I've met St. John the Apostle, a patient that swallowed a cross to have God be "within," a Prophet carrying Jesus for the last four years and now, a woman in restraints screaming with a flow of holy water streaming across her face. At one point she turned her head to the side and sang Christmas carols. Christmas was a religious holiday so it did fit in with everything. And to think that today I found out that my co-worker attends bible meetings most nights of the week because she is a Jehovah's Witness. Not quite sure what that was, but the image of a knock at the door and a poor person spouting God's love and will seemed to be something along the lines of wrong. I had seen too many religious zealots living in the ward to not think that religion was something seriously wrong.

October 10, 2008 – THE HIH PITCH: WE CAN GET YOU CIGARETTES!!

It has been several weeks since my training had ended and I was on my own. In the beginning I didn't quite understand the HIH program. As time went along I began to learn more about HIH. HIH was a big chunk of my job. It was a program to assist patients when they were discharged from the hospital, and it was my job to introduce the program to the patients. It was like pitching a Hollywood studio the next high concept moneymaking movie that sounded too good to pass up.
"I want to talk with you about a program for you once you leave." We sat in the dining room on plastic food break and I handed him the flyer. He flipped it over in his hands.
"Do I read it?"
"Yeah." I pointed to the bullet points that I always did because 100% of the time no one reads it and if anything I wanted them to read the points of help like getting meds, or counseling, or a place to stay. It even suggests help getting a job, which always threw me off because that was what every patient dreamed of and wanted so would agree to the program, not knowing that getting a job was the last thing they would be able to attain, and that would happen way down the road. If at all. I started the pitch.
"It's a program that is voluntary and there for you 24/7…like if you need your medication or housing or a place to go or treatment." It

always sounded so flighty and stupid and not something I would buy at a 99 cent store for 98 cents.

"Can they get my cigarettes?"

"They can help you do that." Total lie. I had no idea if they would get him cigarettes.

"My mom came by and gave me some cigarettes before but she hasn't been back to see me and give me any more." Sometimes the mind would meander, and the conversation would open itself to other streams of thought, which was fine, but I needed him to focus.

"So the program. I'm going to put your paperwork in and see what I can do." He slowly pulled his tired hands away from the center of the table and sat back.

"OK." It was not a sigh and not a thrilled response to my effort to pitch a program that I knew he needed but knew it sounded ridiculous coming out of my mouth. It would just be so much simpler if one of the bullet points on the flimsy flyer said in big fun letters: WE CAN GET YOU CIGARETTES!! Then we would have an excited starting point to get a patient activated in the system and get them back on their feet. WE CAN GET YOU CIGARETTES!! Five words in print on the front of the flyer would work wonders. And why not? Why shouldn't they get their Goddamn cigarettes? It was a negotiating starting point on a long road to getting a life back and away from a dark room with a dirty bed and a moaning scared person sleeping beside you.

HIH made me a salesperson. Sometimes patients changed their malleable mind when I made it sound like they were lucky if they were "accepted" into the program.

"I'll see what I can do and submit your paperwork, but, just so you know… (here I could add a psychological twist to the pitch to get their attention, just so *you* know)… there are no guarantees that they will accept you into their program cause not everyone qualifies, and a LOT of people are on a waiting list and want HIH but unfortunately there are only so many slots out there." This sample pitch was followed by a sudo reassuring look that said I will do my best and kept them maybe wanting more. But it was the truth. The program had slow slots and the patient would have to be interviewed to see if they were accepted only after they qualified for the services. There were so many levels to make a connection to the program and I was at the forefront of it all. I was the first one to approach the patient and explain the program, then find a way to present the case to HIH so they would even consider coming out to see the patient, then I had to get the patient ready which was a full blown pep talk prior to the interview with the HIH rep.

"HIH is going to be here in an hour, you ready?!" Yeah!! Sometimes it was met with a slow roll off the bed, other times, a spunky pounce off the tiles with the teasing thought that there was a way out and someone there to find you shoes. I sat in on the interview as the mediator to help further explain the benefits of the program, then I would follow up with the patient to see what they thought then had to report back to HIH on the patient's interest level and that report was solely up to my discretion in thoughts, words, attitude and style.

"Sure, he's totally excited about the program. Let's move forward and see what kind of housing we can get him." When really 10 minutes ago I was sitting in front of a ghost sideswiped by a random interviewer speaking Gaelic cause she was woken up after an Ativan nap and didn't have her ears on straight yet to understand much so mistfully reacted to the whole idea BUT I still had an orange chance to try and find another time to approach the person and plug the program. Maybe after smoke break when they've had some bird filled air and some oxygen reinstalled in their suffocated brains I could find a new way to pull out the sunset sun from the deep blue sea.

I continually found myself finding ways to approach a person and quickly figure out what I needed to say to try and get them to understand HIH. I searched my mind for buzzwords on the bounce or ways to explain a program that maybe they would like, need, want. Cigarettes would often dart out of my mouth as a means to grab some attention. Cigarettes were crucial to patients and their future stories.

Later that following week I learned about a new rule imposed on the patients locked at Top. There was no, zero, cigarette breaks for any of the patients. Zero. The system had already taken away their life, freedom, and pursuit of happiness. What's next? Water?

October 11, 2008 – THE ROTATING DOOR

I got a call from my office headquarters today asking about a patient who was recently discharged from Ocean and was now at another county hospital. They wanted to know why he was let go. Well, he wasn't conserved and had the right to move onto the next block. Probably next to Street Corner who wanted to return to her bench on Avenue A and Avenue B; however, she agreed to have some follow up with HIH. Not that once she was there she would recall our conversation about having outside assistance, but at least there was a slight chance she'd be helped. Maybe when she came back to the hospital through the rotating door she would reconsider using the program to help her help herself. It was only a clock ticking before she would be off that corner and back in the psych ER. Tick tock. Tick tock.

And they always do. The rotating door only got worse when the county instigated the Code. The Code Kick 'Em to the Curb started up and all but no more than usual hell broke loose. The Code was a way for the county to save money. Or at least that's what it looked like on the spreadsheets made somewhere in someone's cubicle over Shasta from the vending machine. The Code was simple: the psych ER was overcrowded so patients in the inpatient unit would have to be discharged to allow psych ER patients to rotate in. Every day two patients were identified to be ready to go. Well, the ones that were not kicking and screaming. The drugged out snail walking ones were usually the target cause they hadn't done anything wrong to keep them there, but, how can you toss out a fight when you have no energy to punch the air? So once the ER was too heavy full of madness the Code was called and the discharge planner would jump upto the phone and call Mountain View. Mountain View was a place for the Code patients to go. It had a bed and open walls. Patients would be discharged there and out by half past a minute. Out back into the world and back in the psych ER by half past an hour.

Now THAT'S saving the county money.

TOOTHPASTE

She didn't have toothpaste on her face
It was Noxzema.

"I think she can go."
The doctor states
"She has toothpaste on her face. No one thinks that's a problem?..."
The other doctor spouted
"Ah, well…she can go."

I spoke to Toothpaste when she was ready to go
She had some white cream on her face
With pounds of makeup on it.

And she told me she was excited to go
She wore a hat with red and black stripes
A long denim skirt
And fake brown contacts.

She was more than ready to walk out
All put together
With Noxzema on her face.

She was ready to go.

CHAPTER 8

JOURNAL ENTRY - MANHATTAN SUMMER - 1998

I left England no better off than when I landed, except I was 10 pounds lighter and ready to spend the summer in New York. I was back in the sling, a subletee in Harlem, and working at a mergers and acquisitions firm with way too much time on my hands. Being back from my European excuse for a semester abroad for painting character and experience on my face, I decided to keep a journal to keep track of my life, my thoughts and feelings, and did my best to forget my romance abroad with Carter. I made the stupid mistake of letting myself fall in love with my best friend/soon to be roommate my senior year. We had a warm romance abroad and decided, he decided, at the opening of my first and last loving heart, we should just be friends. I went along with the plan because I didn't have a choice. Even though…he was the one who confessed his love for me in the basement of a pub in London, and he was the one that hung on that bleeding heart for weeeeks thereafter, he was the one who wrote me a love letter with all the universe of his thoughts sprinkled on the page, and he was the one to end it. We were going to share a suite with our friends Simon and John so we, I mean he, thought it was best to keep our cool and remain friends. But I knew it wasn't over. But everyone knows that when you sleep with your best friend, everything changes. I wish I had had the wisdom to know that at the time. And, like any girl in the post rejection stage, or any girl wanting to escape the pain of silence and feelings of what the fuck, I busted my ass to get in shape while obsessing over food, fat and weight. Slim Fast blended with ice took front row next to Tanqueray and Tonic.

The journal I kept of that summer in 1998 reeked with a mirror of passages that screamed: You are some sort of insane. And all the answers to all the problems I endured for years could have been realized a long time ago if I would have taken time to read my own world. I wouldn't have to read between the lines. Hypomania was in every word in every sentence in every passage on the page.

June 16, 1998

I am trying to live an honest life but the more honest I am, it seems the more difficulties I find. When one is open and exposed they are left in an extremely vulnerable state, where anyone or anything can affect the condition of that state.

June 21, 1998

I am going through something strange right now in my life, and I wish I could pinpoint what exactly my problem is. 'Problem' is not the correct word, but I am short of any other word. I am alone a lot and I know that is not safe or healthy but, simultaneously, I have no desire to surround myself with people or places. I went to a chic bar on East 53rd and 3rd with some friends that have graduated and work in the city now and it was fun seeing them and catching up, but the whole scene was not so grand. I always thought being young and single in a city like New York would be wild, adventurous and fun, but instead, I find myself talking to drunk suits and ties. That's all they are, Wall Street boys and victims of the ladder.

June 25, 1998

I was so adamant about being in New York for the summer, and swore that I wouldn't spend another summer in Los Angeles, but right now L.A. doesn't sound so bad. I think my family thinks I don't like them, but I just needed to be away and.. I don't know. I am on the verge of tears and long for my old friends, maybe even my old life.

My roommate thinks I have obsessive-compulsive disorder and so do I. He gave me some Ritalin which I do take when I feel like I need them. There, I said it! I am not fucked up or anything, but a little hyper and out of control sometimes. It doesn't make me a retard or incapable by any means, in fact, I am highly functional. I am going to psych services in the fall and will see someone to learn more about it, or me. I am not ashamed, just uneasy about telling anyone.

June 30, 1998

I am at work and totally bored. I've realized that the amount of time it takes me to do a task takes an hour and they expect it in four or five hours. I'm not working on speed but it seems that I can complete work at such an accelerated pace that I have pretty much all day to screw around and even *then* they think I work fast. Boredom is my biggest problem and I fear this is going to slowly kill my spirit, and my brain There is only so much boredom a person can take.

July 3, 1998

Well, I have returned into the abyss of self-denial and betrayal and I feel like ass. I wish I could explain it but I can't even explain it to myself. One of these days my brain will stop causing so many problems and I will be free from my mind. Yeah, right. I am sad that the summer of my dreams is almost over and the reality of life is waiting to hit me in the jaw. I take for granted that I work in a great area and live in a sweet apartment in Spanish Harlem. I guess those material things are nothing compared to the loneliness I feel in this city. I still love NYC, but I wish I had someone to relish the plethora of places available to someone young and energetic. My roommate left today for England for some girl and I am forced to live alone for the next three weeks which scares the shit out of me, but maybe it won't be too bad.

July 4, 1998

I spent the Fourth of July alone making garlic with chicken meaning literally garlic…with some chicken. Like everything in my life I only took things to the extreme. It made me sick. Eating cloves of garlic is like early steam engines riding throughout the night. I was uncomfortably sick all night and through the next morning but still managed to suck back my slim fast blended with ice and was good to go…running.

July 12, 1998

Summer is lonely, but a healthy lonely where I am learning about myself. I guess if you spend a lot of time with yourself, and not by yourself, you are bound to unbind some bindness.

July 15, 1998

Today I had another epiphany. The duality that fights in the soul is golden and realized through my heart, my brain, and my passion. That's what I know, that is all I know, and some of what I understand. I have to love myself and embrace the black and white forces paradoxically confusing me, yet intricate to my nature, my being.

July 21, 1998

I made a new friend today. I was sitting in my ridiculous cube, bored out of my mind, and looked up for salvation. Angela, a tall, exotic, young black woman was standing across the aisle dropping off mail on someone's desk. I reached out to her like a child making friends with someone in the sand box.
"Hey Angela." She turned and rested her arm against my desk.
"Do you have a nightlife?" I asked.
"Ah…no."
"Well, tonight that's gonna change."
And just like that, my summer began. Every night we hit the scene hard.

Dancing, boozing, jointing. No one could stop us. Every club, bar, party, there was no stopping the black and white cookie. It was the perfect set up. Our work hours were twelve noon to seven so we could roll in by noon, hit up the company buffet, guzzle Snapple all day, change in the bathroom at night, than hit the scene all over again.

It was the summer I became New York. Like most, it didn't swallow me whole, it just took bites here and there. Every morning I woke up swearing to my grave that I would not go out, but the devil would take over and I would find myself unable to say no. I refused to go home and be alone, so spent almost every night out on the scene hitting on men like they were band-aids for my self-destructive behavior. I ended the summer ready to go back to the Utopian walls of academia that would consume my life and end the boredom that was the straitjacket of my summer.

Little did I know I was walking back into the gates of my senior year in college headed for a major mental break. I was stuck in a suite with my three best friends. One of them was Carter and we were definitely not going to be just friends, ever.

CHAPTER 9

October 15, 2008 – CRACKSTEROIDS

I have an office downtown in the hood. It had contracts with all the IMI's and enriched board and care facilities so they were in charge of placing a patient upon discharge. My office was The Office on cracksteroids. It was actually worse than the NBC show The Office. No joke. Every time you entered you had to sign in on a board outside the boss's door. You had to sign out when you left or when you went to take a shit. I had a half desk that I shared with another co-worker which was fine with me because it gave me an excuse to spend most of my time in the field. I usually ended up doing my work in the kitchen which I didn't mind either because I figured if they didn't have space for me then I wasn't expected to be there like the rest of the rice stuck together in a bowl. It was mostly Asian because the boss thought they worked harder than other races so publicly announced that Asians were superior. I think the real reason the boss tended to promote Asians was because they would probably jump rope every morning to make sure when the boss asked them to jump, they could actually get some air under their shoes. They were afraid of the boss, and even more afraid of forgetting to sign out when they went to lunch. God forbid. God forbid.

October 16, 2008 – TRADER JOES

TRADER JOES

Trader Joes was generous
And more put together
Than others
On the catwalk
In the locked
Psych ward
That were head hanging lampposts
Staring at the traffic walking by.

Trader Joes had tangled long stringy white hair with a dry scalp and very dry skin.

"It feels like there's tape on my arm." She pointed to her arm between the elbow and shoulder and I wondered how she could feel that when all her skin was peeling at the seams and dripping dust across her nightgown.

"What's your name?" I sat down and pulled myself up. I turned to a young girl with a dirty blond bob and lazy eyes that could barely focus that rolled side by side and in and out and of the back of her head.

"Overdosed." She was too melted down to turn her head to face me, but half turned it to get the words out.

OVERDOSED

She smiled inside
Tired insides
Which resulted in a slight lip movement.

October 17, 2008 – MORE AND MORE MEDS

Medded Out on the 2nd floor wanted to go. She sat in a green chair across the room from a guy slouched in a chair mumbling to his feet while the Cambodian TB positive 61-year-old floated by.

"I have to leave LA." She was serious.

"Where are you going?"

"I'm going to the South."

"Do you know someone there?"

"I have to get out of LA. The lights. The street. Too much going on. I was raped before I got here and now I am here and I don't want to be here."

"I understand that, but I don't have any say in you getting out, your doctor will help you with that." My answer to almost everything. The patients expected something and wanted answers and I wasn't any answer to the ongoing waterfall of the same question with the same pipe running up the fountain to refill that answer with the same water. And I made that clear every time. It took the pressure off for them to try and be a certain way; "ready", "healthy", "totally fine." With me they didn't have to care because I was no one to them. I couldn't get them out, I couldn't change their meds, and I couldn't stop their meds. To some, and not all, I was just a worthless face. To others, I was someone to talk to and pass the time with or maybe try to enjoy it. I was a virtue and a vice. I was a sure way to break down the wall because I wasn't going to change their meds or give them freedom. I was a medical caseworker and that answer always left empty defeated eyes. I didn't even know what that meant. It sounded so technical and was far from the truth of what I actually did, or what I was to these people on a face-to-face, word to word basis of human exchange.

"Where is my doctor?" She wasn't having any of it. I was a zero and she wanted the doctor. "I have a court date on Monday and I'm not sure what it's for or what I have to say to get out of here, or if I should go…" I swallowed my hated ignorance with a pissed off tongue and spewed truth as sad as ignorance can be truth.

"I don't know. I will have to check on that for you."

"But don't tell them it's me that wants to know, I don't want them keeping me here longer."

"I won't." I wouldn't say a word.

"You find out and tell me." She was not stupid. She had a mother…

"She's on drugs." And a father she never knew from South LA. She was tired of the lights and tired of sitting in that chair.

"I have to get out of here so I can stop taking Depakote."

"You have to take your meds if you want to get out of here."

"It makes me sleepy. I get in my bed with the lights on and I'm out for a day and night into the next day. I had a friend in a board and care and she told me about when she had to take meds and how it made her knocked out. I don't like it."

Her eyes weren't as bad as Overdosed upstairs but her mind was right enough to realize that the drugs were too much. The echoes of rounds resonated in my mind as I thought about the ever changing list of meds and the residents that would look up to the doctors to give them the OK, good job, yeah do that, pat on the back without any wait, I don't think she needs that much. And as far as I could tell, she didn't need much, or at least *that* much.

Erica Loberg

IS HE SLEEPING?

He walked over to the chair in front of me and sat down
Grunted
What'ss howsss
He tried some words
How are you?
I asked
Youurr shoesss

He was severely sedated
As he fell into himself
In a chair
By a table
Wood and strong
And lights bulbing
From the white fluorescent scene
Is He Sleeping?

Is he sleeping?
The nurse asked
Are you sleeping?
I repeated
As he sat there
Resting his head
Into his neck
And slowly his eyes rolled to the side of acknowledgment.

October 20, 2008 - IT ALL CAME DOWN TO A LOAF OF BLACK BREAD

I sat down at Trader Joe's bedside and she showed me her list of things she needed to do. It was an organized outline with cursive writing with a sharpie pen that was more legible than anything I could put together with such a thick pen.

I want to see my kitties

I have to clean my room

I want to....

And the list went on with pragmatic activities. We talked about cooking squash and I told her I tried to cook it and made a mess.
"Did you burn down your kitchen?" she asked and I managed a grandma smile.
"No. Just made it too buttery." She told me of a lamb she cooked with too much spice and I laughed because too much spice to her would be a tidal wave of spice to her if she were to enter my kitchen.
"You can have my hair brush when I'm gone." Trader Joe's latest zonked roommate pointed to her hairbrush.
"They never told me I could have a brush, and my hair is so ratted and bad." She strung her brittle skin fingers through her crying old hair.
"You can go to the nurses' station and ask for one, or have mine." Zonked was generous and more put together than others that were head hanging lampposts staring at the traffic walking by.
"So, Trader Joes, how did you get here?"
"I was shopping at Trader Joes for black bread."
"Black bread? I didn't know they had black bread at Trader Joes."
"It's next to the white bread. I wanted the black bread and she called the police and told on me and..."
"Who called the police?"
"That woman in the store. She said I was yelling and called the police." She leaned down on the side of her tape feeling arm and dabbed her swollen deep eyes with an old Kleenex, then reached to the box next to the brush and whipped her eyes with a fresh leaf.

"And what did you do?"

"I did nothing. I should have gone to Vons and get white bread there. I just wanted that black bread."

"So then what happened?"

"So then I'm here, and I swear this place is making me crazier than usual." Than usual. Perfect words of someone observing themselves enough to know themselves. She was worried about her cats, and the social worker had been to her house where piles of shit were all over the place and the cats were hidden.

"When bad people come to my house my cats hide." Another woman who shared the room with Trader Joes and Zonked was new to the ward. She walked in talking nonsense about New York being a bad place and....I blocked her out. There is only so much attention you can give a rambling rude when you are in a conversation with a tired crying woman sinking across her own bed with Zonked sitting up with her motionless face and blank eyes watching.

"She told me my sister was dead..." Trader Joes pointed to her other roommate and grabbed more Kleenex to dab her sandpaper skin around pockets of swollen tears.

"She's crazy, don't listen to her." OK. Not the best thing to say, given the circumstances. What else could I say?

"When I saw a shadow I thought it was my sister. I know this place is making me crazier." Trader Joes was dying to go home to her cats. Her only connection to the outside world while she was stuck inside a coca cola bottle of loneliness. Trader Joes was trying to survive alone in her old age, crippled with her illness, and lost inside terrible independent loneliness. But she knew something 100% clear.

"That's my life story" she sat up and said.

"It all came down to a loaf of black bread."

Later that day I went home to my empty apartment. It didn't feel alone. I guess I had gotten so used to being alone it was normal. I was grateful I made it through the times when I was first alone. When I had no one and nothing to bring me to find a place inside that was OK with having no one. Nothing. Zero. At least I think I was, but maybe I had become so accustomed to it that it didn't matter anymore. Maybe those years early on in my life, lost in my disease, I had training wheels that set me up to only know alone.

CHAPTER 10

JOURNAL ENTRY – MANHATTAN - 1999

Getting my apartment seemed fun, until I was actually there, all alone in a room with a futon and a bookshelf. So this was the life. This was freedom. Living in a box with no comforting distraction like a TV to pass the time or make white noise. I am in my apartment and I am totally alone. I am so lonely that I got a call from a solicitor trying to get me to switch telephone providers and I found myself asking him where he was calling from, how his job was going....pretty much anything I could to keep him on the phone so I didn't have to be alone.

I sat on my fire escape and watched the naked guy across the street and wondered what it would be like to get my kicks out of sticking my dick out the window while watching innocent victims on the street pass by. I wondered if that would cure my terrible deep-seated sadness for companionship and be an end to my slow time. Usually I would stay out till I was exhausted enough to hopefully get by with a necessary pillow for a slim night, but tonight I am sitting here and am not comfortable in my own space. I decided to call my drug dealer and get some marijuana delivered.

"Hi. My name is Erica and I live on 177 East 77th street and I would like to RSVP for the party."

I hung up and felt relief that I would come across someone other than my naked masturbator across the street or some random solicitor. Twenty minutes later I opened the door to my delivery guy and realized he too had other places to go that night; other people to help escape from their sober lives. I sat on the hard wood floor and smoked the pot out of the shitty joint that I never seemed to know how to make. Moments later I was numb. Numb to anxiety, loneliness, caring. I didn't think any more about anything and could stop the ongoing thrust of thought running through my head. Thank God for that.

One puff and the thoughts bursting on and on in my brain were silenced, at least until tomorrow.

CHAPTER 11

November 20, 2008 – THANKSGIVING BY THE BATHROOM

It was Thanksgiving on the ward and the patients sat around a long table in the hallway ready for their turkey, with a scotch taped up banner smiling Happy Thanksgiving written in crayons across the wall.

"I'm sitting at a table...in the middle of the hallway...next to the men's bathroom." Candy was smart, pretty and better enough to be over it and know her observations were true. She was sitting in a hallway with the rest of her inmates ready for their dinner.

"Can I have some candy?" Another patient addressed Candy. She turned to me and told me her grandmother brought her a bag of candy and everyone bothered her for some of it all the time. The patient beside her kept turning to her with his mouth watering open. He was new and fresh on the drugs overdosing his blood and changing the saliva in his mouth.

January 29, 2009 – DEODORANT

DEODORANT

Deodorant needed perfume
And deodorant
For her dreads
Streaming outside her skull
Half baked and nonsensically fried
Underneath her shower cap
I told her I got her some deodorant
And she rolled over in her bed
Friskily happy
Ready for
It
Standing up

Ready
Can't wait to get it
And picked up her soft
Pink pants
Lost beneath her deep belly
And walked to the nurses station
It was there waiting for her.

Deodorant wanted deodorant and perfume. She had her hearing tomorrow and wanted to look presentable. Why shouldn't she? It's only her life sentence to look forward to and apparently it would be based on her hair and nails and standing voice. It was more about presentation than a chart, maybe. At least to her. So she wanted perfume and smelled my Chanel and I said I'd try to get her something, knowing I had some spare deodorant in a cupboard below the stove at home. Some Dove, which I hate and was happy to give her. She also wanted a wig and pulled off her shower cap to reveal sad dry heavy dreads sprouting out of her scalp thick and wondering when they could breathe. At least they weren't lice infested like the last wig on the ward that fell off a bed when a patient turned over in her sleep during her 20-day nap. SPLASH. And the lice tried to flee the scene so bad that they had to evacuate that side of the ward. But they didn't evacuate the TB positives all that fast, if they could catch them through the psych ER that is. I began to wonder how patients could get transferred from the psych ER to the inpatient ward without getting screened for lice and TB. Lice and TB. I'll take lice in my hair over black pipes in my chest. Deodorant just wanted some hair. She slowly pulled down her shower cap and looked up and said, "I just need a wig, I can't go like this." She pulled her fingers through her tired stiff stalks and didn't even know that she was going to be conserved anyway. Her sister and husband weren't going to be there. But the public guardian was. And that was enough. And it wasn't until the next day I realized that the story of what will happen is always a story, even to Deodorant. She thought she was going to some place near Santa Clara to live in section 8 housing when she was really heading for a locked facility filled with slothful feet walking aimlessly across soiled boards on grounds with passersby wondering why they were wanting that next thing without knowing what was really outside. Because there was no outside.

I never heard the word conservatorship when I first came to the hospital. Conservatorship was dualfold. Either you were conserved by the Public Guardian, aka the PG, or a private conservator, aka a brother, mother, blood relative. It meant you had someone else calling the shots. You had someone deciding your destiny as far as where you would go and when you would go was concerned. It required a court and a judge and a reasonable reason for having a person give up their inalienable rights as an individual and have someone else become that God that initially gave everyone the right of free will which was now taken away and given to another person. There was no free will when you were conserved. Your first amendment in the bible, God gave us free will, was taken away. Game over.

The ladder to the nut rag started at 72 hours. It was called a 5150, which meant the person could stay in the hospital for up to 3 days for being gravely disabled, a danger to others, or a danger to self. After those 72 hours the patient could go, unless they still met one of the three pillars of incarceration. After the initial 72 hour hold the remaining steps were deciphered in front of a judge based on a good day, a bad day, a poor response to meds forced upon you or a shitty roommate that caused you to piss on the floor. How you presented yourself that day, what kind of liberal or conservative judge you had, what the doctor happened to say about you that specific fragment of time all determined the slow rise to hell.

February 13, 2009 – PREGGERS

When I first met Preggers she was banging at the door demanding to be heard. She should be heard inside the explosion of wild transactions that transpired in the air on the ward. She had an angry lip and a no nonsense this is what I want and I know the name of the person that has all the answers type of mind.

"Doctor!…Doctor!"

He let her in for an interview which was for once not a podium of people watching the insane and hearing a story about their crippled mind interpreting the world, and for once Preggers was in charge of these asshole Socratic ideological bullshit wandering residents. Thank God. With a capital G. She knew the hospital drill. She had been there before and before before. She could give a wide eye if she was in the hot seat that would be like melting into a plastic stream of tell me everything about why you are here and what did you do and do you think you have a problem. Go…fuck..yourself… is what Preggers would have said given the opportunity. But she didn't because she was smarter than those that put people in a chair to learn about the mentally ill. Stick your dick on a seat and see what the women have to say about it. Stick your ugly birthmark on the table and let us dissect the colors and geometrical shapes and SEE HOW YOU LIKE IT!

Telling people you're mental in front of a stage of strangers must suck. But telling someone you know and love, my father, for the first time was a whole other can of tears.

CHAPTER 12

JOURNAL ENTRY – PARENTAL BREAKTHROUGH MOMENT - 2005

I finally had the conversation with my dad. He already knew about it and asked me if I was shrunk yet. I told him I was still shrinking. I ended up hanging up unfulfilled with my argument or truth on my desperation, so I sent an email. I knew he would get it the next morning, but didn't think he would call me right after he read it.

"Huggums, I got your email."

I tried to sound like I was not still in bed, 10 am was early for me. He was so loving and supportive that I choked back tears that hurt to swallow.

"And I want you to know I understand that there are times in people's lives when they need a shrink. Just as long as it's not some Hollywood bullshit."

The tears dissipated faster than they came. Does he really think I'm some Hollywood cliché?

I had told my dad in the email that I was a miserable person, unhappy in all aspects of my life, socially, professionally, spiritually (I never actually said God or put God in the equation for fear of sounding keshie as my dad called it.) He was in good spirits and took my spoonful piles of mud down his tender throat better than I expected.

"It's not that I am suicidal or anything, I just hate myself."

I was surprised to hear the assertive confident sentences about the terrible state of my mental health verbalized. Bottom line, he's more than a reasonable person with a loving mind capable of supporting challenging times. He made me feel at ease when I told him that I couldn't even answer my phone.

I doubt he'll give me shit for not picking up any time in the permanent future. But it wasn't his fault. He didn't know what it was or how to react because manic depression is a silenced shadow. An unspoken truth that can't be avoided even though everyone tries to, most of the time.

CHAPTER 13

February 14, 2009 - PREGGERS

Preggers walked the halls in her Hawaiian dress with a pink flower stuck behind her ear. You could not avoid her presence. She wore an angry face and held a loud smile.

"I need to make a phone call." She stood at the nurse's station demanding to use the phone.

"Not now Preggers. You already made a call."

"I know, but I need to make another one." There were other patients waiting to use the phone at the nurse's station and there was a pay phone in the dining room. It would randomly ring for patients who had people calling them. Not everyone had quarters, so relied on the nursing phone which always had people waiting. Quarters ran dry for the most part but those that managed to hold onto a few could make calls to their boyfriend, their mom, or someone not really there.

"But I need to call somebody." Preggers was getting nowhere.

"Hi." I smiled. She turned to face me and her eyes popped up.

"Ahhh, you're pretty."

"Thank you. What's going on?"

"I'm trying to make a phone call."

"Other people need to use the phone."

"Please back away." The nurses needed space from the giant colors sprawled across Preggers' obese body. She had already had five abortions in her short lifetime and was pregnant, again. But you wouldn't know that by looking at her because the weight was everywhere.

"Come on. Let's go back to your room." I escorted her back to her room and said, like I always did, "I'll come visit you later." Little did I know later would be later and she would be the first person in my life on the ward.

February 23, 2009 – NOT COLLEGE ROOMMATES

I was having trouble placing Preggers. She was being referred to an enriched board and care, which turned to a referral for an IMI, and now she was on the path to Sunny Side. She had too many bad incidents that caused her to move up the crazy chain so there was no hope in having an open setting. Her bad notes were even a problem at the highest level. Sunny Side wasn't interested. She had been there before and they had that as a reason to keep her at the ocean bay. On top of that, she had a fight with her roommate, so had to spend some time in seclusion which also didn't help her case. Anyone with seclusion in their notes wasn't going anywhere anytime soon.

"What happened?" I asked. She was fresh off the fight.
"She was fucking with my shit!" Preggers pointed at her roommate who sat still on her bed motionless.
"You aren't going to go anywhere if you can't get along with your roommate."
"But she was fucking with my shit!!"
"It doesn't matter. I can't place you with that behavior." The childlike panic set in her face.
"I'm not going to Sunny Side?" She became more panic-stricken. Preggers wanted to go back to Sunny Side. She said her boyfriend was there.
"No. I didn't say that, but they won't take you if you continue to be a problem."
"OK. I'll be good." Her demeanor changed as her anger deflated. She was getting more pregnant every day and finding her placement was a must for after a certain amount of days she would have to remain in the hospital until she gave birth.

A few weeks later it was too late to discharge Preggers. She was past the pregnancy deadline. The hospital wasn't upset about it though because at this point they wanted her to stay for the duration of her pregnancy. If a patient is acute the hospital wouldn't lose money for those days. When a patient got better and went on administrative days the tune changed. Ocean was an acute psychiatric crisis ward. Not the LA Hotel. So when Sunny Side called to let me know Preggers could be admitted she was just within the time frame to be discharged without having to stay because of her pregnancy.

"We can keep Preggers for the duration of her pregnancy. Let Sunny Side know we are not going to discharge her." After weeks of being hounded to get her out, now, all of a sudden we were going to keep her?

February 25, 2009 – AKA

Colostomy bag was a transsexual with a colostomy bag who I had trouble placing because the facilities didn't know if he would be in a male or female room. He was too old for a sniff. A skilled nursing home was called a sniff. He couldn't manage his colostomy bag on his own so no one would take him. He had been on the ward over 100 days and counting. Colostomy aka John. Sometimes the names were aka and other times if they had no identity or social security number or anything they were John or Jane Doe. People had a name they didn't like so randomly changed it and some didn't know their name. Then you get a patient who won't give you his name because he has a record and doesn't want to go to jail.

"Ha..ha I'm Jerry." He had a pipe taped to his throat from an earlier incident maybe involving a pen speared through his neck...or not. No one knew cause he was Tom, then he was...

"Donald."

"I can't place you without a social security number or some identification." And he knew that.

"Ha..ha..I'm Jesus Christ." He knew he couldn't go anywhere without a solid name and thought the unit was the LA Hotel and he could stay there on the county's caring dime. The bill was weeks high. So you do the math and whip out your wallet while you're at it.

"I'm trying to help you. I can't help you without a name."

"Ha..ha." And then the social worker stepped in.

"This is not a joke. You have taken advantage of the system and this is your last chance to come clean and tell us your name or else we're going to discharge you today." He perked up.

"I don't want to go to the street, I want to go to the beach, I have parties to go to.."

"OK. We're done here."

He was gone for less than a day before he wound up back in the psych ER. He was found naked in an elevator and willing and ready to be taken back to the LA Hotel. But one of the case managers in the ER had an office next to mine and so knew the story behind John Doe. She knew that he was playing us and the system so wouldn't let him be readmitted to the ward. The game was over at Ocean and it was about time. Next stop, Eastside Memorial? St. Joseph's Medical Center? Which one should I hit up next? I'll try West Memorial, I like the food there.

February 27, 2009 – HOSPITAL HIERARCHY

I peeped into the window and saw a blob on the bed.
"Preggers, what's up?" I think I asked in the best way I knew how and her face rolled to the side and she rested on her bun of a hair that she wrapped up tight around her head.
"They all trying to tell me they don't know what's going to happen…where am I going?"
"I don't know."
"My heart is beating so fast. I think it's going to beat out and God will take me."
"Take some deep breaths."
"It's pounding so hard. All the stress before was from the baby and now it is from that stress."

An intern strolled in with a machine to take her blood pressure and Preggers said her heart was a problem and the intern was concerned. I told the intern I could take her to the attending and walked to the doctor and she slightly footed forward into his room and stopped.

"Is that the attending? I just need to talk to the resident." She was afraid of the apparent hierarchy of doctors on the unit. I didn't see the difference. I never saw any title meaning anything other than a person ready to go, to do their job. The doctor never made it seem like I couldn't direct an intern or anyone else to his path and I was grateful, or maybe off on the dynamics of the residential medical sphere totem pole of bullshit. Why is it bullshit? Because you should go to anyone when a woman thinks her heart is pounding too hard.

Preggers made it through the examination and I told her too bad she can't stuff food anymore in her breast because her breasts were so big that she could use them as air pillows. When she was tired, she could just drop her head and have support. I got a little "ah..ha," out of it. Not a laugh, but at least an acknowledgment of a laugh.

March 2, 2009 – OPENING CASES aka CHA CHING

Opening cases was case management aka working with patients to get them discharged aka doing what I do anyway but finding a way to bill for it so your company looks good aka make money money money for the county. Opening cases was the county's way of recouping money that was gone due to the financial crisis. Opening cases was case management for patients. In other words, opening cases was a way to bill for services that I was already providing anyway. It all pissed me off.

"So basically we are opening cases to bill for the county since we are facing a huge financial crisis." It was a statement, not a question. I challenged the district chief of DCH who was also the iron fist that whipped the cracksteroid office with a smile that confused them into thinking she was running a happy ship while meanwhile they were scared to use a paper towel in the kitchen to wipe the milk they spilled by accident so would try to clean it in a oh shit panic with their underwear if they had to.

"Well..no. It's about client care. Making sure the clients get the best care possible." But that's what I've been doing. Spin it, spun it, do it. Even now when the term client spun out of someone's lips it sunk beneath my skin causing a blood boil that threw anger into my brain at an electric speed. THEY ARE PATIENTS. PATIENTS! This is not a law firm OK! Not dime dollars or bills in your brief box. I found out sooner, unfortunately than later, that the newest PCest county term for patient, turned client, was now Consumer. A consumer. What the hell did THAT mean. It sounded like someone who engulfed something down the back of their throat. Eat it, take it in. It sounded like someone that took things. I wasn't going to look it up or anything cause the dictionary doesn't play by the modern non rules of colloquialisms that turn

Webster words to something not so Oxford English.

"So this is about money." I just wanted someone to come out and say it. Why now was it so imperative for us to open cases (provide case management which meant talking with patients and writing down what transpired and the TIME you spend doing that so DCH could get points, dinero, props for making money when money seemed to be squeezed so tight that a Speedo on an elephant would be comfortable).

"OK." There was no point in arguing with a table of numbers dictating good patient treatment when you had a job to do. Little did I know that open cases were going to change everything. It meant digging in deep into the lives of these patients, and little did I know what I was walking into, on the catwalk of the mentally insane.

March 3, 2009 - 26

26

Had hair that was blond on the tips
And half way down her face
Next to deep roots
Inside her skull.

26 wanted milk
Which she drank out of a carton
Like those distributed out in middle school
Or maybe even first grade.

26 said yes
To doing every drug
On my list
A check box
Yes
Yes
Some I didn't know
"What's that?"
"I bought it on the Internet, when I was in rehab."

26 was an open door
Ocean breeze
Simmering on top of deep dark depths of
Cool waters
Stirring inside
The insane.

26. I had to get her consent to talk to me and walked into her room
and called out her name.
"26?"

She bucked up straight and quickly smoothed her less than smooth
hair from her forehead away from her wonderment of what was next
and spoke to me with her eyes, ready to listen.
"I'd like to work with you. I'm not a social worker, or a nurse or
doctor, I'm just here to check in and see how things are going and
work on your discharge plan."

"OK."

And it was that easy. She had been in a dozen hospitals in her 26 year old life and was still open to talking with me. She shuffled into the kitchen dorm-like setting with the refrigerator beaming rancorous sounds.

"How long have you been here?" The social worker opening the case for me asked because I was not licensed to do so.

"26 years." 26 replied.

"In here?" The social worker looked perplexed. She didn't get the quick wit or maybe she and others don't get the way a brain works inside the madness.

"She's been here on the planet for 26 years." I clarified and knew immediately I had an in with 26. She said she was molested by her grandfather, and had been in and out of hospitals and was able to keep a straight face. I liked her. If I had to open cases I would prefer to have someone interesting and honest to exchange dialogue with. I was picking cherries and happy that I wasn't leashed to another patient in the common room reading nothing, watching nothing and standing, or sitting, plain. Plain.

March 6, 2009 – SHE PULLED OUT AN ORANGE

"Whatcha you got there?" I pointed to Preggers's right breast squeezed into a tight shirt. And she pulled out an orange.

"I don't feel like eating the chips anymore. I like the orange." It was the first real happy shock. She weaned herself off potato chips and now had an orange in her chest.

Down the hall was Wandering Eye, who I also opened a case on.

March 7, 2009 – WANDERING EYE

WANDERING EYE

His eye wandered to the left on the right eye
When am I going?

He had colored crayon papers
Perfectly taped to the wall
Beside his bed
And a piece of paper beside his bed
Every night
That read
Where am I going?
When am I going?
He pointed to it
And addressed the questions
Every time
He wanted
An answer
To anything
As he should
He came from prison
Thinking people were pouring water on him
While he slept
To
Moaning in the halls
That were loud enough to travel to people
Outside their doors
And feel a pain
If they knew any pain other than a sore
On their toe.

Wandering Eye wanted to know when he was going. I only had one answer.

"You are on the top of the list to go."

When really there was no top of the list. He was competing for a bed with patients in other county hospitals who were also told they were at the top of some list. The list changed on a daily basis based on non daily occurrences. And he still thought he was going to some place down in I don't know where because it was ruffled in the articulation. He pointed to the wall and had a piece of paper by his head beside his bed. In carefully written crayon it read: Where am I Going. When am I Going. That was all he wanted to know and all any sane person would want to know at this point in life, in a stale white ward with random people coming and going and not knowing when or where your turn was in the passing line of nobodies living in somebody's. Going...where? None of the patients knew, and none of the staff was going to tell them.

AWOL was Wandering Eye's new roommate. I decided to open a case on him.

Erica Loberg

AWOL

AWOL wears a thin Armani shirt
From I'm not sure.

AWOL has one tooth on his bottom gum
One loose tooth
Thin and dark like a tired shuttle.

AWOL washes his hair under the sink
And when he missed a day
He told me.

AWOL told me to go fuck myself when I first met him
He said a truth.
He wanted to get out
Of the ongoing locked doors
He knew what was out there
And what he had to do
To get there.

AWOL had a tiny smile
On one side of
His face
He didn't let it go
Across his entire lips
His life was that harsh
That a full smile was not available.

AWOL knew about cars
He knew how to escape
He knew how to push buttons
On people that don't do well
With pushing of any sort.

AWOL had one honesty
He knew who he was
Even when he was smearing shit on the walls
He knew he was ready to go
Because he wanted his bike
He liked riding on the streets of L.A.

AWOL was special
AWOL was insane
Of the sane.

When I first met AWOL he was stuffed in a corner of the room with a blanket over his head.

"AWOL?"

"I'm not talking to you assholes. I want my stuff back." He had a bike back at Shoreline, the place where he awoled twice to get the heck out.

"So how did you get out?" I asked, hoping he would budge from his cocoon. He jumped out of the bed that he had made for himself in a corner against the wall.

"I pulled the sliding door up and took my stuff in a pillow case and drew a string through it so I could drag it over." He was very excited to tell me the details of his flight for freedom.

"When did you do it?"

"When everyone did their last rounds. I knew when to go." And he did. Twice. He managed to pile tables and chairs and hold a wire in his teeth to carry his bag and get over and out of the place. He animated around the room like an excited delinquent talking about how easy it was to steal a car. Then tears hit his eyes. He wanted to go to Reno or out of the spit hitting staff of his other facilities and had a cap on to hide his tears but his red lower lips pumped vessels that revealed the empty drops.

"I have a Cadillac I made. It was from 1975. It had all the chrome in the front and was like an electric kitty. I made the windshield wipers into a whiskey shot. I had a shot of jack and I could drink when I drove." He tossed his head back to show his luxurious love for it. Wandering Eye came back and was upset that I came to talk to AWOL and spent half an hour talking to him when he was in group. I told him I didn't know when he would be discharged and I was back where I started. Wandering Eye's head was back down on his pillow. Hat on. A wall of pictures on his side of the room was growing from all his time in recreational therapy over the weeks. He pointed to the one paper by his head beside him on the wall again.

"Where am I going. And when am I going."

March 9, 2009 - BLAH

I'm not taking advantage of my surroundings. I'm not depressed. I'm not tired. I'm just blah. I'm not using my craft to show the depth of the world of lives that surround me. The world of those that are locked up, or on the street like champions of crazy.

March 30, 2009 - GONE

Preggers left today. I delivered the news that she was going and she said I was her best friend. I teared up so had to excuse myself before anyone saw. I watched her pack up all her things and she gave me her new headband so that I would remember her. I would always remember her. She never told an honest lie.

March 31, 2009 – DRIED BLOOD ON THE WALL

I reviewed AWOL's chart today and discovered he was a 49-year-old with bipolar disease mixed with some antisocial personality disorder. I went to speak with him about Shoreline and when I asked him about it his eyes teared up and he begged me not to go back there.
"You don't know what it's like there. People walking around naked in a circle around and around."
"I've been to Shoreline. I know it's brutal."
"I can't go back there."
"Well, the good news is you can't, they won't let you back." He seemed pleased but didn't realize that meant he was on a track to Top. No one, no one ever wants to go to Top. But he had already had several code blues and managed to pick his nose enough for it to bleed down his broken face when he was put in seclusion. I wasn't there for it but heard about it the next day.
"AWOL, what's going on?"
"I want out of here."
"I'm working on it but you have to try and behave and not get any more code blues because no one is going to take you or anyone that

has continual code blues." He jumped up, opened his mouth, and wiggled his one single lower tooth. It was his only tooth standing up on his bottom gum.

"They put me in that room over there and tried to smother me. They bashed my head and blood was everywhere. Now my tooth is loose." He wiggled the last straw in his mouth and I put his hand down.

"Who hit you?"

"Those big black guys. I called them niggers and they beat the shit out of me."

"I don't know what to say, I wasn't there."

"You don't believe me?"

"No. I didn't say that, I just don't know what happened because I wasn't there."

"Here, I'll show you, there's still some dried blood on the wall where they beat me." I followed him to the room and he pointed to the blood.

"You see, you see, I told you."

"OK. Let's calm down and go sit down."

"Group time!" The recreational therapist rounded the troops.

"We can chat later."

April 1, 2009 - FAUCETS

"Can I see your book?"

"Sure." AWOL handed me his book and I opened it to the front page. My name was written on the side in black ink next to his doctor's name.

"You put my name in your book."

"Yeah, so I can remember you are here to help me get out of here. I've got to get out of here."

"I know. I am doing my best." He nodded like he kinda believed me but also like he had heard that his whole life and was used to the drill.

"You spelled my name right. Some people spell it with a K." I smiled.

"That's like spelling knife with a k. Why would you spell knife with a k? "

"Yeah, like spelling knife with a k. I don't know." I smiled and gave him back his book. It was a thriller murder mystery and it was the only book he had and so he savored it and tried not to read too much at a time. Soon after, I went to the second floor to see how Faucets was doing. I also opened a case on him. Faucets was a 22-year-old Hispanic boy with no one but a parole officer he was assigned to after spending some time in Twin Towers for grand theft auto. He had been in and out of psych wards, spent some time in jail, and didn't have his whole life ahead of him. I thought to myself, please don't become AWOL. Please God.

"I'm ready to go Friday." He ran straight up to me, ready to go. Apparently he did not understand our last conversation where I explained his discharge would be down the road once the treatment team had him stabilized. His recovery included stopping himself from listening to the voices that told him to cut himself and to turn the water faucets on in the men's room till the bathroom flooded. He had three people hovering around him at all times. One was a man with long hair, the other a man with a beard, and the third was an Indian girl. They had been in his life for quite a while and although he knew they weren't real and would tell himself that, they would always win, causing him to do whatever they would say. Faucets turned on all the water in the men's bathroom later that week and no one could figure out why.

On my way out I passed by the seclusion room. The other 22-year-old on the ward that had ripped his eyeball out in the psych ER was on watch 24/7. A nurse had to sit beside his bed and not take both of her eyes off of him. He didn't recall doing it but woke up one day in restraints and a patch over his eye. He said he wanted some glasses so he could see. It would be a long road to recovery.

April 7, 2009 – PAPER DOLLAR RINGS

AWOL was in better spirits today.

"Have you made any friends?"

"No. Just her over there." He pointed to an Asian woman with a trash bag beside her. She was rolling some magazine paper into some origami mold.

"What's your name?"

"Paper Dollar Rings."

"Hi, I'm Erica."

"I taught her how to make these." AWOL pointed to his rings that circled all his fingers. They were paper rings made out of the little money he had.

"She's made a whole lot of 'em." Paper Dollar Rings stood up and walked over with her trash bag. Inside were enough rings that it would take an army a day to unwrap. The bag was almost full to the top and she sat down and continued to make more.

"She's making a hell of a lot." AWOL seemed to be amused in a good way, like he had helped someone learn how to do something that would keep them busy and pass the time.

"Where are you from?"

"Japan."

"Why are you making so many? My God."

"Japanese copy Americans. They copy everything Americans make." I asked AWOL to show me how to make a paper ring and he did. It didn't turn out right so I ended up crumbling it up and throwing it out. He wrapped his ten-dollar bill ring around his finger with the ten perfectly set in the middle and pointed out all the tens on the paper.

"Ten ten ten ten ten. They are everywhere."

"I never really noticed that." Then things shifted gears.

"Are you going to get me of here?"

"I am doing my best." His eyes stared straight ahead and I wasn't expecting to hear next the words that came out of his mouth.

"You can't help me. But at least you can help me learn more about myself." I half expected him to say that I couldn't help him, but never expected the rest.

April 16, 2009 – FLAMING LIPS

I opened another case today with Flaming Lips. She wanted to go back to an enriched board and care: Apple Road. Apple Road, oh Apple Road. God help me Apple Road...

"I've been in and out of places 30 years. I don't want to go anywhere else but back to Apple Road." Flaming Lips was not well liked on the ward. She had a mouth full of dirty words and liked to throw out darting eyes across the tiles during her steady catwalk talk.

"OK, great. Then when they come here to interview you, you have to tell them you want to go back or else they won't take you." She nodded her head and applied more red lipstick. Apple Road did not want to take her back. She had assaulted a staff member and had a history of being verbally abusive, but Apple Road was contractually obligated to take her back.

"You hit a staff member." The admissions coordinator accused Flaming Lips who sat with her arms folded. It was obvious they did not have the ideal relationship.

"I did not. Rudy hit me." Flaming Lips did not recall her previous outbursts and did not like being accused of such vile behavior.

"I don't like sitting here with you accusing me of something that I didn't do."

"We're not accusing you."

"Yes you are."

"OK, Flaming Lips. I'm not going to fight you on this. But given the circumstances, are you sure you want to come back?" The admissions coordinator held his mean breath.

"Yes. All my things are there."

"Well, according to these letters you don't want to be at Apple Road." The admissions coordinator pulled out a stack of letters written in bright non-stabbing blue marker. They were written upon Flaming Lip's admission to the hospital, before she got on her medication, before she understood what happened to her and what was going on, before she sat on the ward for weeks trying to manage the hardships that accompany a unit with crazy people coming in and out of her life one by one. She took the letters and folded them neatly.

"You can have them, I have copies." He was starting to piss me off. He didn't want to take her back and his manipulative manner was certainly not something you'd want to witness in front of a 47-year-old woman who had been through the system for 30 years.

"Are you sure you want to go back?" All he needed was a no from Flaming Lips and he would get a free get out of jail card and be done with it. He had already asked her again and again and again thinking, hoping, that she would slip and change her mind. The mean letters thrown in her face weren't enough. He had to beat her down with a stick with 'Are you sure you want to go back?' spray painted on it. I stepped in.

"She already said she wants to go back. She has already expressed that to you several times." Flaming Lips sat still with a vacant look on her face that had moist tears collecting on the sides of her eyes.

"Yes. I want to go back." Her voice was small and wheedled down to a string sliding out of her mouth carrying a white flag breathing 'please'.

"OK then." He gave a look like it was not over, it was not okay and somehow he would manage to win and break free from Flaming Lips. I had had more than enough.

"You know, per my conversation with my office, you have to take her back because you did not follow the protocol and allow her three days notice when she was admitted, so I don't even know why we are having this conversation."

"We just want to make sure she will stick to the rules." Again, he turned to Flaming Lips waiting for her to crack. I blessed Jesus for preparing Flaming Lips before the interview.

"You will stick to the rules, go to group, take your meds, and not bother other patients?" Flaming Lips sat silent again. Silent and defeated, yet proudly consistent and lightly persistent.

"Yes."

"Would you be willing to sign an agreement that states you will abide by the rules and if you don't you understand you will have to go?" Pour it on asshole, just keep pouring it on till she suffers just a little more. She took the paper, glanced over it and signed it. She dated it April 16th, 2009. I watched her with the pen and thought to myself: it's my birthday. She is signing her life and pending future and it is dated on my birthday. I'll never forget the look of her signature next to the date. It made me sad that there was some realization that things were not good out there. Things for Flaming Lips were not looking up. She got up to gather what little articles she had with her and began to cry.

"Why do they have to make me feel bad? Saying I did all those horrible things when I was beat and kicked."

"I don't know Flaming Lips, but look at the bright side, you are going back to the place you wanted to go." Some bright side that was going to jump start her being...as she walked down the hall carrying her brown paper bag with her meager belongings. I watched her exit the door and left for the day. Happy Birthday.

April 18, 2009 - GENETICS

I called Preggers at Sunny Side today to say hi. I wanted to know if she still had the fake gold bracelets that she loved too much to not have one from my arm. I remember that day she left and she gave me her new headband so I would remember her too. I thought about that day she wanted me to see her baby, and I walked into a room in the hospital with babies in plastic boxes with tubes across their diaper bellies. These were the babies that were struggling to survive. Preggers's baby was sitting in her mother's lap. Her mother had rainbows on her eye lids and fifteen bracelets that jiggled on her arm, and nails longer than a line to get free ice cream on a hot summer day, and some people still believe that mental disease is not hereditary. Some bipolar people liked pizzazz and dressed like it. They embraced loud colors in fashion and welcomed glitter on their eyelids or feather boas swirled around their neck. I looked at her baby and wondered if manic depression would skip a generation and if the lithium Preggers had the last nine months would have a lasting effect on her baby. Her mom was truly crazy and it was hard to be cordial after all the stories I had heard out of Preggers's crooked teeth.
"Ah...you have perfect teeth." She would say every time I smiled. None of these people ever had braces. Every smile told a different story about their lives. And there sat her Mom, and I thought again about all the stories about all her boyfriends and the boyfriends that would sneak into Preggers's room and sexually abuse her almost every night. Preggers was concrete and raw and had so much bad happen to her that it was no big deal to talk about the sexual abuse that started when she was twelve years old. Her mother walked the earth while Preggers would soon be locked in a facility. And now she had to say goodbye to her baby which was going into foster care that afternoon.
"I've never held a black baby before. This is exciting." I laughed at myself. I remember trying to be upbeat. She laughed her special laugh from the soul of her being and I looked at her baby. She had told me earlier that her baby had freckles like mine and she did but they were black. She said goodbye to her baby and that day I walked with her back to the ward to unlock the unit and re-lock it for her so she could go to her room and look through her baby pictures. Those pictures would be all that she had to remember her

baby by.

"Do you think I will ever see my baby again?"

"Of course..I think so. You just have to stay on your meds and get better and you'll see her again." She looked at me like she didn't know and I didn't know either. I knew nothing about the fate of her baby.

"No. I'm never going to see her again." I recalled her folding her clothes on her bed in a nonchalant manner.

"I don't know Preggers. Maybe she will try and find you some day." Preggers had no reply. She sat down and pulled out her baby pictures. Those pictures were the end. They were all she had. She said goodbye to her baby that day and I was damn lucky to be there. I didn't have any answers to her questions but I was heartbreakingly fortunate to be with her.

Erica Loberg

JOURNAL ENTRY – FAMILY LUNCHEON LOS ANGELES - 2005

"You got it from your mother's side of the family." It came out of my father's mouth before the waiter even put down the chopsticks. He smiled and meant it in a friendly let's break unbreakable ice manner but underneath that comment was a blame game that seemed to free himself from any connection to the connection to mental illness. My mom sat silent. Somehow someone was going to be blamed and it wasn't going to be the Loberg gene stream. I wouldn't change my brain, or switch genes. After everything I've been through, and all the ongoing internal carnal manic magic I've lived in, I'm grateful. I'm not ashamed, unlike the long line waiting for centuries behind a family member suffering from a mental illness.

"Maud"
By Lord Alfred Tennyson
What! am I raging alone as my father raged in his mood?
Must I too creep to the hollow and dash myself down
        and die

It was as awkward as awkward would be given the fact that my parents now had a child that was diagnosed with bipolar II and they came from a generation that really didn't know anything about this condition and if they did, they sure as hell is beneath schizophrenic feet not speak of it.

Later on my mother told me her mother was possibly bipolar. She said she never understood or got along with her mother. She was more or less stuck in a house with a chemically imbalanced parent and exposed to all that comes with the madness inside her mind.

Communicating family history could have been another red flag. Ignorance and shame were monster problems eating at a potential discussion on mental illness. Knowing your blood tree is crucial when discovering moods of the mind. In a culture that tends to hide mental illness, and denies the existence of perturbed blood, we are left with dark tunnels filled with ignorance and family shame. The levels of shame accompanying the mentally ill and families living with a mentally ill member needed to come to an end. A cultural dialogue needed to explode. It would be a starting point to punch through the denial that seemed to be intrinsic to the ignorance and shame embedded in mental illness. I was grateful to have a family that woke-up their eyes and ears to my turbulent world and embrace it. Embrace me. But I believe this is rare.

If we can find a way to drop the shame, we might have a starting point to educate and communicate truths that can only be a springboard for discovering help and producing cultural change.

April 19, 2009 – 20 HOURS OF SLEEP

It was hotter than hell at the hospital today. Usually the wards are a shitty hot mixed with dirty clothes but I was used to it. I was kinda used to it. Sometimes the smell was worse than others. I think there have been maybe two days thus far that when I stepped out of the elevator, the smell didn't penetrate my nose and blow through it upon unlocking the doors. Things were quiet this morning as I made my way to rounds. I forgot that there was exercise class for the patients and walked into the room. It always blew my mind that exercise consisted of standing and waving your arms side to side. The patients would stand in a circle and take tiny steps side to side. Exercise is one of the fundamental things to do to help depression, at least it has been that way for me, and here they were moving side to side, right to left, arms up and down at a I'm just chillin' pace. There was a stationary bike off in a corner of the other ward but I had never seen anyone use it. I didn't even know if it worked, so thought to myself next time I would check it out. One stationary bike from the 80s on the 2nd floor and a stand and sway side-to-side circle of working out in the other. It truly was quite something.
"It's so weird that there is no gym for the patients" I commented out loud to one of the residents.
"We don't even have a gym" he replied. I was appalled. How could he say that when these patients slummed around at a dead mans pace up and down the catwalk. Most of the time they just lay in their beds with a sheet pulled over their heads fast asleep pissing the day away. It was strange that in one of the wards there was so much light, there were no blinds to make any shade and they

managed to remain in their beds, dosing on and off throughout the day. On the other ward, considered the dungeon, there was no light. No curtains or shades to even block the light. There were just dark walls. It was as if they wanted them to waste the day away, and away again tomorrow, sleeping. On the patient sheet it always listed the amount of sleep they would get every night. Usually it ranged from 2.5 hours to 6.0 hours. I wondered why they never calculated the number of hours the patients would sleep throughout the day. It was probably too much trouble, for it would be on and off all day long. Mostly on though, however, the majority of the time when I would walk up to a bed of a dozing patient and call out their name a few times till they stirred awake, they wanted to talk to me. They wanted the company and more times than many, when I left they would always say, "Thanks for talking to me." It was a mantra that never seemed to alter the sad hit of pain I felt when I would walk away. The sincerity in their voices made it impossible not to believe: these patients were lonely. They were isolated in their minds and subject to unwanted sleep throughout their day. I do believe they were over-medicated. I had heard too many slurred tongues, saw too many slow zombie like walks, and too much of the stench of no bathing. Maybe bathing would be too much of a task when you had so little energy. No one wants to splash water on their back when you are half asleep, half dead with no physical signs of wanting to be alive. Especially when it's cold. Depression is an ugly thing and I was reminded of it every day. I feared the day depression would return. I recalled the days it sat inside my retina, and took over my face down to my toes. I still feared the time I endured it. I don't know how I ever did.

CHAPTER 14

December 5, 2007 – STALE BREAD

DECEMBER

I don't want to leave my bed
Because I don't want to dress
I'm not happy with my body
I don't shop
I don't want to enter a room with fluorescent mirrors
Deep ascension into a deeper cycle of self
Hate
The sand falls fast
Darkness engulfs me
I breathe in white air
That turns black in my mouth
Ascending down my throat
Into the abyss of my stomach
A void covers by rolls
Of fat that hide it.

Backwards efficiency.

I wake up after hours, almost a day, of sleeping and roll from my bed to the chair in my living room. I thought dismantling my TV would keep me from falling into a TVpression but now I only watch my one DVD over and over and over to the point that I hope I'll come to be over it and get my ass up and out of my apartment. But I don't. I continue to watch it, and am thankful to have something to watch. My brain is stale bread but not hard. It's just stale, sitting there on the shelf of my head and flat as a pancake. I have no thoughts, no words, no passion, nothing. I thank God I have no phone calls to return because it gives me a panic attack to have to check my messages to hear someone on the other end wanting to know where I am, what I've been "up to." And I can't say absolutely anything because they know. The people left holding onto an absent friend know about me and would think things about my state of mind. I don't want to burden anyone with my sterile world, but maybe that's a lie. I don't want the burden of people knowing and having them think about it, or try and talk to me about it, because no one has any idea what my world is like here stuck in my hollow apartment where the only thing keeping me cognate of some relationship to life is my cat. I wish I could just cry and let it all out so I can be done with this. But I can't. It's worse. I feel nothing but am sure that all the personal pressure to stay on top of my mental state, go running, be productive (whatever the hell that means at this point) which is void is a deep internal long cry that has no end. I went to Santa Barbara to the premiere of my friend's film and drove home with light on my cheeks. I wish I knew what was that thing that made me get up and go. I know I'm scared for myself and the myriad of days and days going by with nothing other than some cheese and a screen. Even preparing my plate of cheese and crackers is doing something that makes me feel alive. So it would be nice to capture whatever made me get in my car and drive in a jar and breathe into it when I am scared again. How does fear lead to strength I'll never know. I was anxious when I was trying to get out of the city mostly because I slept 14 hours and was 6 hours behind my attempt of a schedule. I only spent one night out of the city and actually had someone say I was glowing when I went to my usual local market to get some more cheese. Just that little accomplishment brought some life back into my face.

DEPRESSION IS A BEDROOM WALL

I stare at a wall in my bedroom
And am relieved to find meaning
That I am doing something
I find hope that my next step will be more than hours of watching a wall
Even entertainment in the red paint that gives me a color
To watch.

It's doing something
And it gives me pleasure to know
Although I feel nothing
I am doing an action

When I stare at my bedroom wall.

December 12, 2007 – MOTHERFUCKER

Motherfucker.

I don't want to isolate anyone in my tears of loss. So I have no one to call. It's much worse to scare someone than it is to scare me with my loneliness and tormented activities these past few weeks. I never thought about it before, but now I have a responsibility to the people I love and throw my problems at, I can't do it and have them stress for me because they know I'm fucked up and worry about me every second of it when I actually articulate it. This is why it is better letting it reside in me. I feel better with that than causing my loved ones alert concern.

December 14, 2007 – FAT IS NOT FUN

I have gained weight, WEIGHT, on lithium and can't take it anymore. I come from a family that if you are anorexic, you are doing well.

December 18, 2007 – MAKE THE CUFFS TIGHTER

JAILTIME

I lie on the steel bench

And rest my head on the toilet paper roll.

I don't fit on the deck.

I'll just sleep.

As I lie on a metal shelf that doesn't fit

My body

Like lying on a cement dock

Resting my legs against the wall

And wait.

They took my bra, my shoes and socks, than asked me to remove my necklace.

Everything.

Take everything.

I press the call button

And tell the sheriff

That I need my medicine

Nothing.

I was released a day worse off than before.

I'm in drunk driving school and I'm so lonely that I look forward to every Wednesday night that reeks hell for everyone else. I never, neverrrr, leave my apartment not just because I am fiercely lonely, but also because I am fat. A whole new kind of fat where I don't even recognize my ass anymore. The lithium has taken over my fat and has managed to pump bulge inside my pants, and rolls down my stomach and pushes out of the flesh of my arms. I don't recognize myself. Maybe because it happened so fast. In less than a month I have gained 30 pounds. I woke up one day and I looked like a blow up doll that some hyper air machine pumped up in a matter of seconds and I hate myself. It's bad enough that I come from a family with a long history of eating disorders. So now I can't even see them. I can't even see my own family. It is that bad. But, I have my drunk driving school friends who have never known my skinny self and don't have to know me ever again because NO ONE wants to see ANYONE from that dreaded class where you have to tell your terrible DUI story. I'll admit, my story was bad. Every class the new admission had to start with how they got their DUI. I happened to have a citizen's arrest somewhere in Alhambra. A kid from Jordan pulled me over and asked me if I was OK. I was driving funny. I said I was fine, of course, and went on my way. But he followed me anyway because he was worried. And as he followed me, he called the cops who I later told to make the cuffs tighter when they were already searing my skin. But I didn't know the heavy belt was on his hefty way. And I wasn't sure if he would. So when I was trapped in a cul-de-sac like a rat in a cheese shop with my citizen's keeper behind me, I got out of my car and did what any other normal person would never do. I walked up to him and started making out with him because THAT was the first thing that crossed my mind to get out of this rubbing alcohol mess. Sure. Just walk up to this stranger and start throwing your face in his mouth. That didn't last too long though because the cop showed up. In my defense, I had lowered my meds and was on a manic high. When I told my DUI story everyone was silent. Oh, like YOU'VE never used your sexuality to get out of a jam. Please. But I wasn't about to fess up I was bipolar.

I had enough labels strapped across my chest. Fat and crazy was brimming at the top of the stove I lived on. But the other DUIers were the only ones who knew my story. Only they knew me as fat. So deciding what to wear, putting some mascara on with a swipe of lip-gloss was the first time I've actually gotten ready to face the world with any semblance of I can do this. Well, I had to do this because if I didn't the judge would send me back to jail and there was no way in HELL I was going to spend another night in a cell lying on a dock with my legs up against a metal wall while some tattooed muscled shirtless freak across the way watched me and waited to catch a glimpse of my hovering ass above the old rim while I tried to take a piss. On the positive side, the drunk driving school is a temporary savior from the dark walls of my brain. I must be terribly lonely. Beyond recognition. Three months, six

months, nine-month programs. The people are normal. As normal
as normal is when you are pulled over for racing through a dark
orange light after one and a half beers. Maybe that's why I like it so
much. Regular citizens with families, friends, a life outside of their
DUI.

January 2, 2008 – DESPERATE

It's during times of desperate attempts to find your place in this
world that ideas enter your head like, maybe I should revamp the
dead feminist movement and give it a Botox brow lift. On a serious
tip, I think it's time to discuss what is going on with the deep seated
desperate attempt to land a man, and what that entails, thus giving
insight into how we need to adjust accordingly.

January 5, 2008 - ?

Unemployment proper. Sleep, eat, sleep, feel the head swim in
"what the fuck should I do?"

January 8, 2008 – NATURE VS. NURTURE

Is it nature or nurture. Both. But I lean on nature and the beast that
needs to be tamed. Without emphasis on the beast, it doesn't matter
where you are, you can find a bed to sleep in and not get out of
anywhere. You can also find a night open to gallivant throughout
the streets picking up and talking to whoever crosses your manic
path.

January 15, 2008 – THE ROLLER COASTER RIDE

I've had some pseudo manic nights for the past few weeks. Going
out meeting random guys and taking them home or going home with

them. I'm not having sex but long for a kiss so do that. I did have two boys in my bed at one point and managed not to do anything with either of them but was in the middle with no space on either side to fall apart. Fleeting physical companionship in a night over does make me feel better than no one and I don't think it makes me lonelier in the end. It is something to hold onto and recall in my memory so I know I am not a total recluse. I even started talking to a neighbor a few blocks down and went out to dinner with him and his T-bird friends which I enjoyed. I like throwing myself into other people's social lives and know that I can hold my own socially without exposing the truth about my silent life. I stopped taking my lithium because it made me so fat that I plummeted into a deeper depression. I told my psychiatrist that I would rather be skinny and crazy than fat and sane and I believe most women would say the same. Regular people get depressed for gaining weight so one can only imagine a chemical depression on top of a fat ass. Since I've lost weight I do see a significant difference in how men treat me and it should give me some power but it's more that I don't want to eat. I'm hungry but don't care. In fact, when I do eat I cook so I am having some type of social interaction with something, even if it is food it's something other than just a screen. Food's a living thing, right?

January 16, 2008 – THE LEECH

I know that my younger sister Olivia is onto me and says she can tell I'm manic from my text messages. So, there's another one I have to watch out for. She is the only person in my entire life and journey of shit that is close enough to me and my disease to know when it's taking hold of my existence. She has enough to deal with than to worry about me. And the last thing I need is for her to tell my parents and have them get that whole can of what am I supposed to do opened up all over the sink.

AND BE SMILE

And be smile
Happy
Like time is invented
By man.
Time, thoughts, knowledge, exuberance
Of feeling already or understood?
That's when the pain in your gut cries laughter
And relief pours down your open pores.
Do we know that the known and unknown are the same?

Sloan is in town and I can't even muster the will power to get in my car and meet her for frozen yogurt. I have nothing to report about my life and am ashamed. Plus, I am pretty sure I can't pull off the smiley everything's marvelous and I am full of life and happiness when my eyes are like gray coals sucked into my head as the depression has lodged itself into my sockets and has managed to slowly suck the life out of me like a Goddamn leech.

A SCARY FACE

Crazy eyes
That pump through the air of vision
Watching an unknown
A not so blank state
But a stare of blankness
That's hit with a truth
Out of the head
From the insides

Scary
Face.

Not fear
Not knowing
Pure unknowing of the self
And who that is
Why like that?
Is that me?

"Again and again and again"
By Anne Sexton

I have a black look I do not
like. It is a mask I try on.
I migrate toward it and its frog
sits on my lips and defecates.

I have to do something because death is not a solution. Death is not
a solution, it's that bad. There is no solution. Ache pulls down my
deep throat when I come to realize that death is not a solution. How
fucked up is that? What's left after that? A live death like that
green fluorescent line that screams across the computer shield, runs
horizontally with a ---------song when someone dies. Now that's
death. For me, it's a green vertical line on the screen but you're
alive and standing up. Alive in death. Death is way too scary to
even speak of and I am thrilled that I have no intentions of thinking
about death. But, having said that, living in a coffin, my bed, most
of the day and night, in a funeral home, my quiet apartment, day

Erica Loberg

after day with consciousness of a living death sucks pretty bad too. I just don't care and want the days to melt by so I can wake up and hate myself for wasting another week.

INSIDE THE LIMBS

I'm close to the end.

The end of no ends
Of dark nonsense
Of nothingness
Without any hope
Or productive path
Or desire to
Become what you are
What you need to be
To be alive
To be you
The person sitting here now
Inside the limbs of God's creation.

If only my music was in me so I could dance around my apartment. Music has always saved me in the past and even that is of no interest. Now THAT is the beginning of the end.

I love dusk. It is staring at me in the face and if I move from my chair to the balcony chair I will be forced to be there alone, with myself. The silence of my brain living in the silence of the balcony and sadness that dusk is slowly fading away to night is too depressing so....I'll keep watching my DVD instead.

January 22, 2008 – THIS IS BAD

I decided I needed to get out. If I didn't change my living environment then things would never change. Once again, this decision happened in a speed of a light. My cat almost died and crying outside the vets jumped my mind into the idea that it was time to go. So I found people to sublet my apartment while I temporarily move to New York and when I hung up, I threw my hands in the sky and said, "Yes!" And felt nothing. But at least my body physically responded to the good news even if my internal state of existence is numb. This is some more bad.

January 24, 2008 - DICKWADES

So I stopped by my local pub to get a beverage and started talking to a guy who showed me pics of his daughters and then he had to go because his wife was calling him and he texted me when he was outside, asking me to come out so he could kiss me. I'm not sure why that happened, but if I had a shot of my face when I got that text it would be worth getting it to begin with. Stupid assholes and their dicks and the poor women that screw them.

January 25, 2008 – MEET THE NEIGHBORS WHY DON'T CHA

I am meeting some more neighbors. I was on my way home from my taco bar when I saw a couple on the street open a door to a staircase heading toward a party. I smiled like I was also a party invitee and climbed the stairs to a huge loft full of people drinking and chatting. I made my way to the balcony where I found a nice warm seat by a fire and was immediately hit on by some guy. I told him I would make out with him but not have sex. He wasn't so keen on the idea and I excused myself to go find someone else to talk to. I walked up to a hot guy chilling in the kitchen and the next thing I know we headed toward the bathroom. Clothes flew off our backs as we devoured each other. I felt sexy. I caught a glimpse of myself in the mirror and sure looked sexy. It was just what I needed. Some hot make out time with a hot stranger in a scandalous outpouring of lust all over the bathroom tiles. I walked home feeling refreshed and hit my pillow wondering how I was going to get sex, especially with my no sex rule that was beginning to result in wild outrage that ended with me walking out of someone's bathroom while people in line gave that look, ah, yeah. What I should have done was tell the guy that I was interested in having him as my booty call, no names, no details, just someone to call on a moment's notice for some sex. That kind of sex I can justify because it would be with the same person and a way for me to stop having bursts of why am I doing this no sex thing and is it driving me to insanity moments in the kitchen when I unload my Portobello mushrooms.

At least I still have my vibrator. I even changed the batteries today after trying every way to figure what which way they go. I thought I had just replaced the batteries recently but they were already dead so was thrilled to find it working again once I dropped in some new ones.

January 30, 2008 - CARDS

I realize now when I picked up a few cards on the table by my door that there are more people than I realize that I have interacted with who happen to have significant others early in their relationships. If I had a filing cabinet for every card I've ever received from a man it would be like one of those overstuffed recipe index card holders with all your grandmother's recipes stuffed inside and handwritten by herself with her cursive pen and neatly packaged in a clear plastic covering. Maybe it's because I am thirty that I seem to come across more unavailable men who are in the early stages of a relationship and part of me wants to get in early and try and show them the light of my jazz. The guy's card I hold now was someone from the Santa Barbara film festival who was not my style, but someone who always seemed to be there: in the hotel room chillin' with some actor I was supposed to know, at the bar grabbing his drink, at breakfast next to me, unlike the guy in the bathroom recently who I wanted badly who also had a girlfriend, or the guy from the bar with pictures on his phone wallpaper of his kids that sent me that text about kissing me who I definitely did not want. They all had second date girlfriends and I wasn't interested in two of them but enjoyed their conversation, which means I only wanted the bathroom guy because he was hot so I can't say I am being good at this point. It was all physical. What I want is a hot booty call. I've never wanted that in my life but whatever this was was not working.

Erica Loberg

February 2, 2008 – PORTOBELLO MUSHROOMS

I like to cook Portobello mushroom in Marsela sauce and put them in the oven for two minutes with some shredded Parmesan reggiano from Trader Joes. Anything more than that will burn the top beyond the brown crust you want and pop them in your mouth. It's sad, or maybe funny, how something so passing to most people is just that, passing, to me it's something to do today, tonight, to look forward to, to do to prove that I am still human and can enjoy the act of making food even if I don't want to eat it. Anyone would be thrilled to not want to eat, I mean women and the faggots in my hood, but to me it's another red flag.

IN THE STREAM

I had a nervous breakdown today
At least I think I didn't have it
All together
And then out of nowhere
There was a great idea
Sit in the shower
Sit on the floor
And let the water come down
While you cry
In the stream
It's so much easier
Than whipping away
Tears
Or shutting off your nose
With a quick swipe of a hand
It's cleansing
It's me
Draining into the floor
The plunging persistent
Harsh warm water
Sprinkles down my body
Away from my pain.

I think from now on

When I am depressed
I'll crawl to the bathroom
And turn on the cold
To wake myself up
Out of myself.

February 12, 2008 – THE METAL HOLE

I went for a run for the first time in weeks and came home to my voice huffing and puffing behind let's pretend I'm not tired vocals in the answering machine of my psychiatrist. I sounded OK, at least I think so and was not crying when I said I needed to come in before my scheduled time in two weeks. When he returned my call I was sorting through tulips in Trader Joes with my cart filled with four bags of Parmesan cheese and two packs of Portobello mushrooms, the small ones that you can pop in your mouth instead of the large ones that I was accustomed to, and lowered my head when I heard his voice on the line and he asked if I was OK. OK. And the pump of hungry tears beat at the back of my throat. Actually he asked if I was all right with a pulse in his voice like he was worried that I was not OK, like suicidal or in a bad place to the point where I was in bad company with myself. He even asked me in the meeting the next day if I was suicidal and I was ready for it when I said it would at least be a thought to have versus not having any thoughts at all to the point where I don't even care enough to even care that I don't care. I didn't care about anything; running, or showering or dancing or wandering thoughts or analytical purpose in the trees when I walk by sad people or those that aren't sure why they are blank. Blank is the worst way to be, and that's what I told my psychiatrist today because it takes a trunk to those that want to die and plan something. In the driver's seat you have a choice but in the trunk you have yourself bound and gagged with darkness and no clue as to who or what is keeping you hostage. But at least you are not ready to die but know that you don't know when you will be released from the uncomfortable fetal position you live in inside the metal hole. Of depression.

February 13, 2008 – MORE MANGOS IN THE BATHTUB

I took a bath tonight, the first since my days of eating mangos in the bath tub on East 77th and was stared down by the man with his cork screw eyes and his long nose taking down the water that was above the rim. I put a firming mask on and once I got its frozen pack sealed on my face I smiled at my outrageous yellow walls beating out against the mirror and was pissed. I took the tube of whiting paste and splurged it all over the face pack and sat in the tub washing my mouth periodically to relieve my mouth from the chemical paste of so help me God I have yellow teeth. And then I got out. And I felt good and removed my plastic guard only to save the remaining amount of paste that was probably four times the amount of what I needed and put it in its neon home and smiled. I saw some great results and feared the rest of my diet Sunkist would destroy the chemicals that were still eating at my yellow grinds and took a straw to the matter. It's harder than you think to suck down a sip, gulp, or pour an amount of florescent orange down your cheeks without hurting the white workers at their best to absorb the plastered gel smeared across your franks.

February 14, 2008 - THE SEX CONTROLLING PILL

I saw my psychiatrist today and told him I was staying off the pill because I like feeling like an animal with fierce sexuality and he wanted to make sure I was being safe.

"So you do use condoms right?"

"Yeah." And I did. But I didn't feel comfortable taking about sex with my shrink. I'm not sure why but when he would ask me about my sex drive I tended to avoid the conversation and keep my answers limited to a fine, same, whatever. And when I said I wasn't having any the inevitable would come out.

"Do you pleasure yourself?" The most hated and feared of all questions.

"Yeah, sure." Quick, easy, answer, done. So I never really told him the truth when it came to my sexcapades or the amount of masturbatory behaviors I indulged in. The session neared to its end and he made a point to make the point that he thinks I am at a point where I feel the mania and can go with it or decide to steady myself and I laugh now thinking that there is no way I would NOT dive into the mania and thank God I am not that stale, slow, pathetic, lame, lonely, and tired asshole I was on the swing shift so don't know why anyone wouldn't magnet themselves to the fridge when that's a comfortable place. Fuck that. I am milking the wild excursions as long and hard as I can. I am NOT returning to anything. But I will say I will cut back on my Trileptal because I was twitching at night and the guys I have slept with can feel it and think I am just in a REM sleep when really I am on meds that have long term side effects which sucks because if my brain needs it, it should not have any effects.....but no one seems to have a grip on bipolar minds so we suffer as a result. I've decided I am going to pull back on most of my meds and see if I can utilize my energy for wild accomplishment.

Why would anyone decide to stop a manic delight and pull themselves in? It's not just a release. It's a lease on yourself. Take it and lease it until you can't afford to anymore because you have bad memory. Your mind's on a ride at a water park and you skip words in the middle of sentences when you write. It that fast.

February 15, 2008 – MY HEART FALLS DEEP

My heart falls deep in my gut and on our soft arms under our flesh and when you live like that... with such piercing reality and heart beating with a bat passion, you have to step back. You have to create a barrier...but it's all bullshit. Because regardless of our ability to isolate or pontificate strength...you will always be the weakest.

Everyone knows the most arrogant hard steeled people walking the planet are deeply unaware and conflicted. It is human nature to decide if you are going to bear arms or stand naked. Some that bear arms don't know they are actually lashing out like a frightened beast that knows too little about life, so arm themselves. Others...you cry. We cry a lot and wait for those times when we're not diving deep inside and not aware of everything. Those times when you are free to enjoy life.

Life. It's yours. Perceptions.

February 17, 2008– BRITNEY SPEARS UNDER SIEGE

Britney Spears under siege. E! discussed her behavior as manic. It's hard to tell since she lives under the hills somewhere under the Hollywood sign that may crumble down the mountain at any earthquake moment and beat some natural real life sense into the kitchen. She gives the wrong voice for bipolar disorder.

It takes a pop culture icon to bring a magazine cover "Britney is bipolar" to add to the constant confusion about this unique disease and make it seem a question and a new buzz world. Why do we have to have an E! True Hollywood story to contemplate conditions?

February 18, 2008 – THE DEFINITION OF DEPRESSION

I am searching for cheap therapy since my psychiatrist thinks it is sooo needed for my ANGER and everything else. I'm not angry, I'm pleasantly pissed. I am stuck in a world that doesn't talk to random people in the elevator. I think when my neighbor said I was negative it struck a chord as did some personal attention to my ingestion of information in this world.

So... The term depression is used to describe a persistent sad mood and/or loss of interest or pleasure in most activities.

They forgot to add….you stare at your balcony and wonder why you are not able to crawl to your chair and be alone in the night, when being alone is part of depression but being alone in your dusk is too much. Most activities? There are NO activities and since your activity is watching DVD's then you are actually doing something. It's an activity you enjoy so that's not depression, it's senseless nothingness. This is what they should say as a description:

Depression is a place you are and don't know it is, not you, until you get a line of thought that crosses the blank field that says, ah, this is life and I don't know anything else and so fuck it.

That's it. At least that's what I just came up with, which is good since it is something other than numb fingers on the computer tips.

February 19, 2008 – CODE WORDS

I went to visit Sloan today and she suggested implementing a plan. A code word when things are bad. She is the only friend that has always been persistent to reach out to me and that was beauty. Sheer beauty. I told her I couldn't have her see me like that. Like a blank wasted out face that stares back at me in the mirror when I try to find me. When that's me. You could not ask for a more amazing force in the universe to keep attempting and knowing when to leave a message that states, if you are not talking to anyone just let me know that so I know. And I got optimistic messages from my dad when he was at the beach with the dog in Malibu. And yesterday I was at lunch with my parents and not able to tell them the dark January and now at Sloan's patio table folding my face in my hands as I cry and fight back falling forward because if I do then I will not stop crying because the memory hurts, but more the memory of these people trying to help me, call me, talk about the beach or chipper life.

MY MOM CALLS AND WANTS TO GET OUR TOES DONE

My mom calls and wants to get our toes done
There is no
Fly by the seat of my life
Anymore.
They want to know something
They can't ingest.
Let's go to lunch
They say.
I don't want to be one of those assholes
That says no
Sorry…busy…lie.
Medication saturates my brain
I am eager to appear
Normal
To be
To be.
They try to be somewhere
In my existence
And it's great
In its heart
But it won't give you
A telescope into my unhappiness
I love you
I love you so much.

February 20, 2008 – NORMS ON LA CIENAGA

I got through dinner with my dad without thinking about any big issues and had a good time. We ended up at Norms on La Cienega and had beads thrown on our backs while I slid a chocolate milkshake down my throat and tossed Tabasco on my eggs and left a sausage half knifed so my dad could take the rest and enjoy our time at a diner on La Cienega.

February 21, 2008 – THE SIGNS ARE SCARY

I sat up and felt sick and felt better staring at the ceiling at the bumpy mold, little bumps up and down for a couple hours and remembered what it's like to be depressed. I can't believe I lived though that. And now it seeps in. The signs are scary.

February 27, 2008 – BUBBLE OF KNOWN

Is it that much easier to hate me, than to love me?....At least I know you'll never have apathy, just yet.

Erica

So I sent an email to Carter. And that is my solution to a back alley dripping dirt off the fire escape water that is mine. It's myself and I'm tired of thinking about it or him and not doing or being or saying anything. It's boring, unknown, unplaced and not what we should live for, to be, to be alive, action driven, sweaty, crying, pathetic, lying, expressionless, dirty. Without that why do people even think to stop and drop those inside of their bubble of known?

CHAPTER 15

April 22, 2009 – MICKEY MOUSE

Back on the 9th floor, outside the ocean breeze that smelled through free nostrils, I was ready to go to the doctor's rounds when I opened the door to find filler. I called him Mickey Mouse. He had one of those Mickey Mouse watches with gloves that would point to the time. He was high up on the chain of the authorities of the hospital so that watch threw me off. He was not excited to cover for the doctor and he blew through the updates on the patients. Later that day I was walking home, and saw him drive out of the parking lot in his car. It was a smart car, one of those tiny cars, and it had a license plate that read I heart small cars. I laughed out loud. He was a tall man squished into a tiny car with a Mickey Mouse watch and was above all the attendings. I didn't like him very much. He wasn't present or very friendly the few times I said hi. Today I said hi and he simply walked by. OK, I thought to myself. Go drive to Disneyland. Maybe it will help your inability to be cordial or maybe I intimidated him. He wasn't one to deal with my type of lady. That I knew for sure, and the doctor was on vacation in Asia. It would be interesting to see how he would continue to ignore me. I had a choice to make. Should I not give a shit, blow him off with not even a fake smile? Or should I be kinda generous, with a likable behavior? No. It wasn't me to pretend and lie. I'll just be myself and make decisions extemporaneously as our interaction would continue to unfold.

Later that day I checked my mailbox. I never had fan mail so I don't even know why I asked to have one. I suppose this is a good time to disclose the truth behind my position at the hospital. My company insisted on having DCH liaisons in all of the county hospitals. All county hospitals were run differently and at Ocean, particularly, there was a long history of someone not wanting a liaison and, as a result, that someone made that position difficult for the poor individual that happened to be standing over a bed waiting for a response from a leech stuck to a moth ball. I was the current liaison that happened to be there, and she was out to get me. The

Demon. She was a supervising psychiatric social worker.
"I've had four cigarettes for breakfast and it's not even 10 am." I overheard her say to one of her minions. The Demon was a bitch. A serious manipulative controlling bitch that treated her social work staff like they were queens above the clouds while she pissed on the medical case workers and treated them like puppets that she would push around and intimidate with her mean scorching stare. She was the reason I was moved to the 2nd floor (I had befriended one of her discharge planners that she happened to dislike and separated us as a way to punish her), she was the reason the past 6 liaisons quit within a three month period and she was the reason my life was slowly becoming hell on wheels like the patients that were wheeled into the ward strapped like they were during ECT. She hated my boss and as a result, hated me. She didn't like having an outsider come into her domain and have any say or play any part in any aspects of social work. I knew walking into the position the terrible history of treatment of the DCH liaison but managed to stay low and drive hard despite the passive and ongoing aggressive behavior. She wasn't going to get to me, at least not yet.

April 25, 2009 – LONG FINGERS

The doctor conducted an interview in rounds today with Long Fingers. He was a tall black 20-year-old kid who had been in jail for drug dealing and wound up in the hospital after having some trouble at home.
"Do you know how you got here?" He glanced around the room looking uncomfortable to be there.
"Can you tell me what you remember about how you got here?"
"I met the girl when I was fifteen. I spoke to her when I was thirteen. I spoke with her on my walkie-talkie. She would talk to me on my walkie-talkie." Schizophrenic patients tended to hear people talking to them through the TV or out of a desk drawer. A walkie-talkie at least sounded sorta normal given the other options.
"And then you met her?"
"Yeah, and there were some people. There was this game. My mom and step dad were playing a game."
"What kind of game?" He sat silent.
"I'd rather just talk to you alone instead of in front of all these

people."
"Are the people here now?" He looked confused, as was I. He was talking about all of us and the doctor seemed to miss the boat that anyone, with or without a mental disease, would feel wary of a room full of people staring at them while they sat on display trying to recall why they were now jacked up on meds and stuck in a room with slugs in a bed. It broke my heart to see the look of fear and confusion and I'm not sure what the hell is going on look on his face as his long black fingers rested on his knees.
"There was a ghost. A holy ghost. And my mom was on the phone saying that I was baptized." I wondered if his mom became hysterical when he was talking to a holy ghost and if she was shrieking on the phone about her poor son who had visions of a ghost when he should be saved as a baptized Christian.

April 26, 2009 – 31 YEARS LATER

This morning I sat down in the kitchen with a new patient to talk about his discharge.
"Hi, I'm Erica."
"I'm Rotating Door."
"I want to talk to you about a program called HIH…"
"I don't want HIH."
"OK. But let me explain it."
"I had HIH before, I don't want it."
"When did you have it?"
"About two years ago."
"Really? Where?"
"Hollywood."
"North Hollywood Mental Health?" He scooped his fingers into his eggs that looked like they were scooped out of an ice cream carton with a scooper. His plastic utensils with a clean white napkin rested beside his food inside a plastic bag.
"Would you like me to open your fork for you?"
"No." He continued to dive his fingers into the powder moist eggs and picked up some bacon that didn't look cooked because the white fat was still there like none of it ever saw any cooking heat.
"So you had HIH before and they didn't help?"
"I need to get an ID. I need to get out of here."

"They can help you do that."

"No they can't. They didn't do anything. I just need some bus tokens so I can go to the St. Francis Church."

"You need housing."

"They have housing there, and food." Blah blah blah blah. I was losing an uphill battle. All I had to sell was HIH and apparently he was already in and out of that system. He only lasted a week in the real world.

"OK. Do you have any family?"

"I have a father."

"Where is he?"

"Compton. I just met him." He opened his apple juice and took a gulp, finishing off the baby carton sized box.

"When?"

"Here. He came here."

"Well that's nice. So you have him to help you." Rotating Door kept the same face with no sign of excitement, sadness or wonder and finished his meal.

"It has been 31 years and I met him here for the first time last week."

"Well, if your dad's not going to take you back you need some kind of outside support when you leave."

"Naa. I'm going back to the church."

"You sure you don't want HIH? You get free therapy! It's something."

"No, I'm cool." You can't make someone get help no more than you can make a family member give help. But sometimes the reality of life makes you do something. Anything. Even when you think you can handle it all alone.

April 26, 2009 – NO TOUCHING

Later that day I went up to the 9th floor to give an HIH brochure to Long Fingers. I entered his room and he was standing staring straight out at the view. It was a beautiful view. He turned around and had dead eyes and a faded air outside his face.

"Long Fingers, I want to talk with you about a program for you once you leave." I handed him the flyer and he flipped it over in his hands.

"Do I read it?"

"Yeah." I pointed to the bullet points that I always did cause 100% of the time no one reads them and if anything I wanted them to read the points of help like getting meds, or counseling, or a place to stay.

"Can I touch you?" He tried to put his arm around my waist and I turned away from him as a nurse walked into the room.

"No touching!" Long Fingers was startled. He stood back. I left the flyer on his nightstand next to his bible. The bible that he told me he would open randomly and read a passage that would help him.

"Thanks for telling me that."

"That's fine. Read about the program and I'll come back tomorrow if you have any questions."

"No. Thanks for telling me you can't touch people. I didn't know you couldn't touch people."

Back down on the 2nd floor I walked into the unit to leave a Rolling Stone magazine for the patients. I walked into the nurse's station to ask one of the nurses where I should leave it. The Lioness was one of the head nurses on the 2nd floor. She was in her 60s and sat inside the nurse's station like the mother of her den. She was the kind of woman that would sit up proud and treated the ward like it was her domain. She was busy on the phone. I turned and found Clozaril.

"Clozaril, how are you feeling?"

"I don't hear any voices."

"That's good. The Clozaril..."

"Clozaril." I was surprised he could pronounce the word.

"Yes, so it has stopped the voices, that's good." He nodded his head.

"So drawing that blood once a week is definitely not worse than hearing the voices, right?" He nodded again. I realized I was still holding my Rolling Stone magazine and handed it to him.

"Here. You want to read this?" He took it in his hands and flipped through the pages.

"Just make sure you share it when you're done so other people can enjoy it." I don't know if he heard me because he was one with the book as he strolled away with it.

I walked away thinking about the days I had to go to a clinic in

Beverly Hills to get the lithium levels in my blood checked. Every time I went there I was reminded that lithium was a metal. A metal beating on my brain and melting my blood.

April 27, 2009 – SKID MARKS

"I tried to kill myself." Skid Marks thrust her wrists in my face so fast and hard I almost got some of the dried blood on my forehead. She stood at the nurse's station showing off her wrists that had thin recent slash marks from some instrument that was fine as a needle.
"Look! See, I tried to kill myself. I slashed my wrists." She was happy to be there, proud of her suicide marks. I recalled a medical caseworker warning me a few days ago about a patient in the ER that thought the ward was the LA Hotel. She liked to show her bloody wrists to people. Did she like to commit suicide for attention? Or was she lonely and had nowhere else to go so would slice her wrists to get a roommate on the ward? Or maybe she didn't know what she wanted or why she did it or how to stop.

Skid Marks was a heavy woman. She had a tendency to sway when she stood and even now sat off her center of gravity. She had been at a board and care but was tossed out for destroying a soap dispenser. It was the reoccurring theme that accidents would happen in the confines of a board and care and no one was there but the patient and the soap dispenser so who's to say who did what. The soap dispenser always wins. She told me she slipped in the shower and tried to hold onto the soap dispenser to avoid falling and they didn't believe her. But if a place didn't want you, it only took one thing that might have happened to knock you out to the wind. Skid Marks had a tendency to reappear in the ER. She would cut her wrists to get readmitted and I asked her about that.
"Do you cut yourself because you wanted to, or to get out?"
"I cut myself to get out of the board and care." She said she cut herself so she could come back because she had nowhere else to go. She was at Burger King and ordered a whopper and small fries and had some money left to use the bathroom.
"You have to buy something to use the bathroom because the bathroom is money operated." She told me she stayed in there 15 minutes, pulled out a razor and cut herself to get out. She said she

left the bathroom and there was blood all over her blouse from Wal-Mart. She said when the ambulance came with the police they "way overdid it." And that it was a "waste of taxpayers' money." Now she was here and she was pissed cause she was on Level B which means no smoke break.

"My room is clean." And I looked around and it was.

"When I'm rejected I give up. So no shower, no more groups, no more doing nothing. I'll brush my teeth because I love to eat but that's it. Dr. K destroyed my trust today." Dr. K was a young obnoxious resident on the case. It was easy to lose with Skid Marks, but it was hard to see why it wasn't easy after all the shit she had been through. She was like so many of the patients that thanked me when I spoke with them and Skid Marks was almost ready for anyone to walk away and knew the drill. I told her I had to go and she took it better than her initial distraught behavior in the hall. I waited for her to look at me, recognize me.

"I'm Erica." She nodded.

"Erica." And her face never lifted from her swinging neck. Her eyes never left wandering right to left across the tiles while she spoke and periodically whip the clumps of middle to dry spit off her lip with her nightgown. Skid Marks wanted to go back to Top. She would rather be locked up than be at a board and care that she could wander out of, end up at a Burger King for a whopper and fries, and then found bleeding in a bathroom that required a quarter.

April 28, 2009 – BIPOLAR II

I came across my first hypomanic patient today and read his chart. Upon admission he said he wanted to sleep and never wake up. He took 100 sleeping pills and ended up in the psych ER. It was noted in his chart that he said "I see no light at the end of the tunnel." He was the first bipolar II patient I had come across in the ten months I had been there. Was it the suicide attempt that got him admitted? Did he really want to kill himself, or could he just not take the restless blazing eyeballs any more and needed a God damn good nights sleep? I wondered about the dark tunnel quote and if that ever filled my eyes. I also just started stopping my Wellbutrin a couple days ago so I could sleep better. It seemed to work so far. Next stop…lower my Lamictal mood stabilizer…?

DEEP THROAT

And then I remember that I haven't taken
My meds.
And I run to the cupboard
Quick knock back
With a deep swallow
And it's still stuck in my throat.
Resting.

Now sitting in the back of my throat.

You still need to take it.

Later I walked into rounds. I was the first one there as usual and the woman with scabies and a white eyeball with a hint of blue shade so embedded in a thick white shield it was hard to believe there was an eye under there, asked me for a piece of paper. I handed her a piece from my spiral and asked her what the paper was for.
"I'm writing the mall."
"What for?"
"I want them to send me some make-up." She folded the paper evenly and placed it in her purse beside her fashion magazine.
"What are you going to ask for, lipstick?" I smiled.
"Maybe." She strolled out and the rest of the treatment team incrementally wandered in for the doctor's table. After rounds I went to see Skid Marks. I started to speak to her and was interrupted by another patient.
"Can't you see I'm speaking to her right now?" Skid Marks belted out. Getting one on one attention in this place was a luxury which was evident in her response.
"I'll talk to you later." I smiled at the patient knowing that later may never be later. After talking with Skid Marks for five minutes, I too had to go.
"Fine, just go." She obviously had a strong past of people walking away from her mid her time to talk. I took a step back from my time and offered her to come sit down on her bed for a chat. She told me she wanted to go back to Top. Top, the holy God please don't send me there Top. She refused to go back to the board and care and preferred Top. It was all ass backward. Then I though about how Sunny Side, a sub acute, was ten times better than an

enriched board and care and that was better than a regular board and care so it all kinda made sense. She told me she didn't like her roommate at the board and care and they would blame her for things she didn't do like break the soap dispenser in the shower.

Later I did another HIH referral. Landscaper thought he was going home Monday but the family wasn't sure if they wanted him. He threw a potted plant at his brother-in-law. He told me he was in the family landscaping business and he thought he was going home to do some planting. I told him I couldn't keep a plant alive if my life depended on it. I couldn't seem to figure out if I was putting too much water or too little water in the pot. He cracked a smile. I was told the social worker rule was to not share anything about your life or experiences in life. I understood that ideology but I wasn't a social worker so that rule didn't apply to me.

JOURNAL ENTRY - FALL SENIOR YEAR CAN KISS MY ASS – 1998

After a summer of silence the moment had come.

"Hey." He turned around and had a bottle of Tanqueray in his hands. I reached forward to give him a hug and got a stiff plank. I knew this moment would come with a scared look in his eyes which couldn't handle it.

"Tanqueray and tonic. My summer drink."

"Yeah right." He couldn't stand the fact that we currently liked the same drink. Maybe it reminded him of the day he picked me up at the train station for John's 21st birthday party in a broken down church in Oxford and we were both wearing a pink shirt.

"How was your summer?"

"Good." He walked to the register, paid for the booze, and walked out the door. I followed him pretending our first encounter after months of what the hell happened with us, and what is going to happen to us, was just fine. Everything would be just fine. I kept telling myself not knowing how much everything was not going to be anywhere near just fine. We were on the beginning of a road that would tear ball down a hot tunnel to hell. A hell unlike I've ever known that would be an on and off nightmare stinking in cloudy love. Ready, set, fuckkkk..

School started and classes were coupled with heightened anxiety. I practiced Ashtanga Yoga all summer long to help release the consistent anxiousness that possessed every second of my existence, and now I found it hard to juggle five classes and find time to practice yoga as much. The pulsating anxiety along with the question "What are you going to do when you graduate?" wasn't helping much either. I felt like saying in response, please go fuck yourself. I am 22 years old and have no idea so back off. Unfortunately, that answer was not acceptable. It seemed that the entire world was centered on getting that first perfect job out of college. All the Wall Street boys were dropping resumes at Goldman Sachs, Morgan Stanley, Chase Bank. You name it, and I didn't live it. But, I engulfed it in the apartment I shared with three Wall Street bound boys. Simon had Goldman and every other bank whoring themselves out to get him. John had to choose between the first and second ranked investment companies on Wall Street, and Carter, my old best friend turned European lover, turned into one of the biggest nightmares of my fragile life was also headed to Wall Street. When he returned he took everything back. He said he was delusional and lonely in Paris and just used me to fill the void. He said I was crazy and deranged. I was the crazy one. A word that would continue to haunt my life like a sick dog tag.

Crazy.

He said he never loved me and that there was no way in hell he ever would. I was devastated but also thought it was all a lie. I thought he was deluding himself with poison in his horns and he did love me but couldn't take it. But that didn't help my living situation which resulted in daily painful agony and no one to turn to.

Being an English major, I was in denial that I was fucked. There seemed to be only two jobs available for my English ass: a teacher, or, I could fill a cubicle in some big-ass office, pushing papers and making spreadsheets for the big guy chillin' on his yacht smoking cigars, catching marlin and making a few "business" calls while the helmsman stirred the ship. Yeah, well, no thanks. Don't get me wrong, I interviewed for everything: advertising, publishing, public relations... You name it. But none of it was for me. Or maybe I wasn't for them. I wasn't the best interviewer in the world because my answers to their mundane questions were not so mundane. They were honest and that sure doesn't get anyone far in this world. I don't even know what I said that was wrong but it always ended in a bizarre look across the table and an "OK, thanks for coming in today." I was stuck in a suite full of over-achievers who knew exactly where they were headed, and had the means to get there, and I was left clueless and scared in my room alone while blasting Help! by the Beatles. And that chummy '"You can do it" fake smile across my face, trying to pretend I had it all figured out and was not stressed at all, was fading, fast. I also looked like a dyke in a suit.

I played the music at a high volume in my room trying to write a cover letter and spice up my resume for the sixth company I was to interview with, Mathews Advertising. A knock at my door saved me from the formula letter I was writing.

"Do you need help?" It was Carter.

"No. But you do."

"No seriously, what are you doing?"

"What are you doing?"

"I am trying to study. Is my music too loud?"

"No. I just thought I would take a break."

"Well have a seat. This is the first time you have entered my room on amicable terms." It was the first time Carter walked past the threshold more than a foot or so. It was weird. For a revolting second, I felt the normalcy that was blasted in memories.

"So how is the powder baby wipes?" Carter was dating one of the Johnson and Johnson heiresses.

"What?"

"Amanda."

"Fine."

"Good."

"What do you think of her?"

"I am not going to answer that."

"Why not?" He sat at the edge of my bed waiting anxiously for my response.

"Because."

"Fine. It's not like your opinion matters."

"Then why do you ask for it?"

"I was just curious."

"Yeah, right. Whatever."

"Well, it has been real, as always."

"Yeah, real shit."

"What?"

"Nothing." He got up and left and the Beatles sang my heart "No one I think is in my tree. I mean it must be high or low." I was sick of my high and low. I was lost. I was desperate. I was going to take a step toward help.

The next day I sat in psych services ready to find an answer to end the worst year of my life. God, please don't let anyone I know walk through this lobby and witness my inability to slap on a smile and choose a career today!

"Ms. Loberg?" The receptionist had to blare out my name in front of everyone waiting.

"Ah, yes, right here." Fuck it. I stood up tall and proud. Hell yeah, I want some medication and someone to talk to. I walked into a tiny room and was faced with my "help." A tall thin weasel man in his early thirties sat behind a desk.

"You must be Erica."

"Yeah." I sat down and crossed my arms and legs, refusing to relax.

"What brought you here today?" Here goes everything.

"Well you see I am a senior…never been in therapy before by the way…and I have no idea what to do for the rest of my life or where to go or who will listen and I have no one to talk to."

"What about friends? Do you have any close friends?" What if I didn't? He knew nothing about therapy. That question could be grounds for suicide, but thankfully, I had plenty of friends.

"Of course I have friends."

"Do you talk to them about your worries?"

"Yes, sort of." What did this bifocal kid, who probably lived a life of nerddom, know about anything. I was a second semester senior about to face the real world in a few short months. I had serious roommate problems, no job and anxiety attacks about the future.

"Do you take any drugs?"

"Like weed?" From his reaction I could tell that he wasn't asking about recreational drugs, nor was he prepared for the truth.

"Sure, I smoke weed, on occasion." The lies felt good. They masked the pretentious judgment I felt searing my skin.

"But you do other drugs as well?"

"No. I don't even smoke weed that much. Only when I am with certain friends."

We baked it, smoked it, boiled it on the stove with butter and poured it onto toast for breakfast. Ryan. Simply put, he was hot. I could enter his suite filled with five other roommates, and swim through the haze of bud to find him ripping a bong hit like we were at PCU. What started as a few joints here and there turned into a daily fest for me to calm the anxious panic of my brain. Plus, there was always the potential that Ryan would hook up with me. I would enter the boys' suite and everyone would chant "Give her her medicine." They thought I had way too much energy and couldn't handle my excessive enthusiasm. Bong hits rolled to giant blunts which resulted in munchies which ended in pot brownies. I was a pothead. But it was okay because I never bought it. These guys grew it right there in their closets.

Pot, booze, plus..and..what?.. ok…there were nights I lost the connection between my body and mind and thought to myself, this is it. I have intoxicated myself with enough escapes and now it is time. I closed my eyes and prayed to God I would return from the complete lost of mind and body. The world was blank, and I was sure God was pissed.

"One one thousand. Two two thousand. Three three thousand." OK, I can still count, even though I can't stand up, or even cry, but I can count. I didn't want to die without realizing that something inside of me was choosing to do so.

The nerd continued to stare me down.

"Okay. So there are no other drugs being used."

"I have tried Ritalin. Actually Ritalin is something that a friend recommended for my hyperactivity and inability to sit still, which was really hard to start taking because I hate the idea of taking a drug to alter the personality that God gave you. Like all those kids that are on Ritalin because kindergarten teachers can't deal with their innate energy. Maybe they should return to the old days when they would simply strap kids to their chairs and not let anyone out, you know?" He didn't know.

"I see. Well, your time is up. Would you like to schedule another meeting? I would like to explore more and talk a little about your family life."

"Sure, why not." I stood up ready to leave this ignoramus.

Fresh cold air hit my face. I thought I would go back. I never did.

CHAPTER 16

April 29, 2009 – LARGE BUT NOT IN CHARGE

I experience my first live attempt at an awol today. For some reason I never seemed to catch those that made a run for it. There was a guy that ran and did a jump kick and was able to blast through the doors. He spent his life on steroids so had it in him. Then there was a guy that hovered by the door waiting. Waiting for someone to make the mistake of not checking out the mirrors before entering. He did a side sweep out the door but couldn't figure out how to get downstairs so wandered to the east wing of the floor. But today I was the one waiting by the door watching a 500 plus pound agitated man pacing back and forth in front of it. He was a new admission. The staff carefully tried to get him to walk away from the door while they waited for the code blue staff to arrive. One of the nurses was the only one to stand at the front of the crew with his white gloves on trying to calm the Large but not in Charge gown. Then one of the other staff appeared with a plate of food. Eggs, bacon and a blueberry muffin.

"You want some breakfast? You have to come over here to get it." It was like using a treat to bait a dog but worse. He started to edge toward the nurse holding the plate of food. The nurse slowly backed up into the seclusion room with the food and Large but not in Charge decided it wasn't worth it. He backed away from the staff and went back to the door. I decided to go around the back way so I could get to my quarter office. By the time I got there and stepped outside the code blue team was there, eight of them. It took eight big strong men to get Large but not in Charge in restraints while he mumbled "Mommy, Mommy" all the way.

Later on the 2nd floor I wandered down the unit and Eyeball came up to me. She was sporting my Kate Hudson in Almost Famous knock off jacket with the feather looking boa around her neck. I couldn't believe it. She looked marvelous.

"I like your new coat." She smiled. Over the past few weeks I had donated a bunch of clothing to the patients.

"Thank you." She did a little twirl. Later the nursing staff said the new clothes really helped her feel better. Her behavior was much better and she seemed to be more stable. I always thought that clothes really didn't matter but looking at her now sauntering down the hall she seemed confident. Her clothes did make her feel better on the inside and that mattered. If anywhere it mattered here on the unit. I was lost in thought when the normal attire breezed by me. A frumpy nightgown with splotches of dirt, piss and shit stained into it with loose fitting socks. That night I put together another bag of clothes. The rule was if I had not worn it in months, someone else could wear it tomorrow.

SWEAT PANTS

It's not like I am depressed
I still get out of bed
When the sun's not so conquering.
So what if I want to wear
Sweat pants
Every day.
I'm just bored, OK.

April 30, 2009 – TOP MUZZLE

I got the email today that AWOL was going to Top come Monday. Just like that. He wasn't streamlined but got there really fast. And he was the most acceptable man in the unit. He no longer needed time out when he took his medication to make sure he ingested it and not puke it up or cheek it. He was a silent wonder patient not bothering anyone like he did originally when he was referred to Top, and now he was Top. He was going there despite his behavior the last sevenfold weeks. They always look at the last two weeks of notes to determine the level of care necessary for placement. He didn't want to go back to Shoreline which was a lower level of care, meaning more random people wandering the halls mumbling words across the walls without any knowledge of the next step forward to a brain to distinguish the rest. AWOL was no idiot. He knew that all he had was bad and that bad was in levels of badness. However, he just might like Top like Skid Marks. But there was one primal problem. The cigarettes. Since cigarette breaks were banned for the staff and the patients so help them God, I would think that the norm would be go fuck yourself now, which was the sentiment AWOL had when he got here and I have yet to tell him he's leaving. I am not sure I can tell him the news but I am. I am. I didn't. I didn't get a chance to because he was shipped off over the weekend, so I was too late.

May 6, 2009 – THE TRUE YOGI

It was actual yoga time on the 2nd floor. After my bitching about the lack of physical activity on the 9th floor, I was pleasurably overwhelmed to see that yoga was happening in the common room. The psychologist on the unit was pulling her legs and arms out to do the warrior pose and did it right there with everyone else. And she was interested. They watched the video of a man on some cliff in the desert while the sun went down enough to make that orange glistening effect on the scene and they paid attention. It was great. I was so impressed, relieved and happy. The best part was when I saw one of the patients lying on the floor flat and pressed into the gray tiles. She was lying straight like a stingray among the yogi practitioners and it was like a dead person lying there out of nowhere. She lay there still and chilled. The true yogi stance of them all.

May 10, 2009 - DETROIT

DETROIT

Detroit was a young black kid
His family was from Texas
Maybe
I think
At least he said they were
And he shook my hand like a regular kid.

I gave him my Eminem book
And he flipped it over
In his hands

And saw the price tag
40 dollars
WOOHA 40 Dollars!
Like it was Christmas on Sunday with an Easter bunny jacked up on
coke
And I said he could have it
And he took it
And the next day he gave it back to me
I read it
I read it all
He said
And he turned it over
In his hands and said he read it
In one night
Because he thought it was a loan
And I said it was a gift
And he stood quiet
Not believing
And I walked away
Speechless
He spent one night in this hellhole crazy place
Blazing though a book
Just to get it back to me
When it was his forever
Not a sentence he heard
Or never understood

He read it in one night.

CHAPTER 17

May 20, 2009 – MORE FLAMING LIPS

Flaming Lips was back. I walked onto the 2nd floor.
"What happened?" A brief smile crossed her angry cheeks. Cheeks of recognition of someone she knew and liked.
"What are you doing here?" she asked with more of a smile.
"No…what are *you* doing here?"
"I need to have my cigarettes."
"I'm not in charge of that. The nurses will help you with that." She became disgruntled in a quick switch of disappointment and I took a deep breath and asked her what happened, again.
"AWOL owes me two million and six dollars."
"Really."
"Yes. I gave him two million dollar bills and six single bills. Is he still here?"
"No. He left a couple weeks ago." Meanwhile, I'm wondering if she knew she was in a different dark ward on the 2nd floor and both of them were originally on the 9th floor where light would be a problem for a vampire.
"He owes me two million dollar bills and six dollar bills" she reiterated.
"For what?"
"I bought tobacco cigarettes from him. I bought six rolled cigarettes off of him and he owes me change."
"Where did he have that?"
"In his backpack."
"Oh…"
"Can you just change my board to an A? I've been here for 24 hours. They have to change my name to an A." She pointed to the board hanging in the nurse's station with all the names of the patients and there she was: 49C Flaming Lips with a big bold red B beside her name. Flaming Lips knew more than I did about the nursing board where they wrote down A B C for the grade you have to get to get a cigarette break. She was fixated on her good behavior and that mark beside her name matched her scarlet letter behavior.
"I'm not in charge of that."
"Oh." She backed off for a moment then was back in her zone of I

need to get a cigarette. I knew from now to who knows when she would come to me to get whatever she needed because I was the one that got her off of the 9th floor and made it possible to get her in Apple Road. And her 5150 intake read the same thing. Kicking staff...verbally abusive..they were looking for a reason to get her back at the hospital and out of their lives. I went through her chart and saw that behavioral plan that she signed a few weeks ago after a grueling session of queries that occurred to try and make her slip up and not be re-admitted to the joint. I found her dotted line signature that she signed in front of me and knew. This was not her fault. Or if anything it was a fault waiting to happen. The outside world was waiting for her to slip and get pissed off enough to make a ruckus and get her back in the ER. And now she was my patient, again. Just like a lot of them that rotated through the locked doors.

Rotating Door was also back. He had been discharged two days before returning to the psych ER. He laughed upon my entry into his room. I asked him what happened and how he ended up back here. He said he went to the church that we planned on going to for shelter and food and they weren't having it. He bought some coke and ended up walking really far to his not really sure where I'm going place and ended up here. I asked him what actually happened to make him end up back at the hospital and he didn't want to talk about it. With a laughing smile he lay down in his bed straight like a funny child and I pressed him to tell me more and he simply said nothing.

"So you bought some coke?"

"Yeah."

"And where did you get it?"

"Ha ha from.." He was not going to finish the sentence.

"OK. I don't care where you got it but tell me what happened after you got it."

"I don't know." He said it with a smile in the air above him.

"OK. You don't have to tell me. But I want to know what happened with your father."

"He visited me."

"He visited you here?" I was surprised after the initial first encounter on the 2nd floor that he actually remained in his life. It was refreshing. Even though he was not willing to take him in, he was there in the smelly sick ward to visit a son he'd only known for a couple weeks or so.

"Yeah. He came here to see how I was doing."

"Well that's awesome. So how did it go?"

"Fine. " He continued to smear a smile across his face, looking above at the silent white wall in his free jail cell, and held the same sentiment that he had the last time I asked him about his dad. It was a whatever. No big deal. He was going to be left out alone when he was "stabilized" even though he was apparently stabilized a week ago on the 2nd floor. He would probably not ever see his dad outside of the hospital. That was the non-irony of the situation. It was pure why. I pressed him some more to tell me about the time between his coke usage and what unfolded after and he smiled and again said he couldn't tell me.

"I'll come back later and we'll talk." He smiled that I'm not necessarily pulling a fast one on you but I'm peeved about being here and will say what I want and do whatever the fuck I want. OK. OK.

Back downstairs Flaming Lips had on some new lipstick that was enough to stop traffic. Her beaming red flames outside her face drawing up into the face of anyone in her space made any room look mundane.

"When am I getting out of here?"

"I'm still working on it."

"I want to go to a board and care. Is that going to happen?"

"I put your paperwork in and so don't worry. You'll probably go there." Probably meaning a safe raft on the ocean of unknowing what lies beneath. I didn't know and she sure didn't know and it all seemed so arbitrary. It seemed a good day or a bad day on the outsider's part to make a decision about the fate of someone's life the following year, or even more. It was that temperamental and hard to digest.

CHAPTER 18

JOURNAL ENTRY - MANHATTAN MAY – 1999

I managed to graduate. I ended up walking alone because I was totally estranged from my roommates who were my best friends for four years. After months of tormented fights with Carter and lost hope of closed dreams, I ended up moving out a month before school ended. I moved into another senior dorm on campus and tried to start over with new friends and I was left alone in my shoebox room with Cervantes carved on the side of the library outside my window. I remained close friends with Ryan, thank God, but losing all my previous four years of existence with friends off my freshman floor was rough. It was rough sand to attempt to do my best to surge ahead despite the wave of loneliness tumbling down on me while I swam on top of the sand at the bottom of the break. Carter and I weren't talking and the guys ended up taking his side so that was that. We had had an I don't have a word for it senior year and now it was time to enter the dreaded new world. I found an apartment on the Upper East Side and began my life. Little did I know my life was headed for a manic *in* depression.

JOURNAL ENTRY - MANHATTAN SUMMER - 1999

"Which one do you want?"
"I don't know, I don't care, which one do you want?"
"I like the one in the Donna Karan personally."
"I knew you would. He's already talking to me, so, do you want to instigate the pass off?"
"Sure."

I always found women's bathroom talk interesting. Almost as interesting as them trying to mask taking a bowel movement by playing with the toilet dispenser, faking a coughing fit, or flushing the toilet a few times when a crap is about to hit the water tub. I wedged myself in between the two girls at the sink and quickly washed my hands. I exited the bathroom and searched the room for

Angela. She was living in Brooklyn and we managed to stay friends that senior year and now we were back living in the city enjoying life together. The club was booming. Angela and I walked around and scoped out the crowd.

"Let's get drinks." We wrestled our way to the bar and smiled at the bartender.

"What can I get you girls?" He was cute, not hot, but cute enough to be a bartender in New York.

"I'll have a martini and…" I looked at Angela.

"Red wine please." We got our drinks and chilled at the bar.

"I'm tired of hitting on guys" I complained to Angela.

"Then don't; I don't."

"Yea, but there are so many cowards in this town. I don't get it."

"Maybe if you showed some patience."

"I don't know what that is." And I didn't. I never would.

Several hours later, I stumbled home, convinced I was walking a straight line, as my mind raced through the events of the night. I climbed the four floors to my apartment and managed to make some concoction of tuna fish, tomatoes and pasta, which I wolfed down before I hit the hay.

ALL THE TIME

I walk home
Alone.
I hear voices.
It's not kill kill
Or die.
It's think think
Thoughts thoughts
All over every
Non-dead moment.

It doesn't matter
Who it is or where it comes from
It matters when it talks
And says your thoughts
All   the   time.

Everything you see
Everything you feel
Everything you are
Everything inside has a voice
That doesn't shut up.

And my feet hurt
I bend over and fix the strap of my shoe
And the band-aid is crushed beneath the strap
I stride through the discomfort.
Is this my crucifixion?

And my journal entries continued to pour a skyscraper of the truths of my mental disease pumping in my brain. My brain was living in a hypomanic world that would slide off the page, or jump into my ears.

JOURNAL ENTRY 1999

I am exhilarated and lonely. I am living in a studio in NY and it is very strange because I never thought it would result in profound loneliness, however, that explains why girls glue themselves to that one guy if they happen to meet him. Dependency, that is the problem. Girls are taught to be more dependent than any boys so they manage to put all their marbles into one bag, or one ball sack. I want a ball sack.

Life outside of college is interesting. Every day is a new diet mixed with an old obsession with food, fat and my body. I am sick and tired about obsessing about my stomach, my thighs and whether or not I have a defined anklebone, but that doesn't seem to change the fact that I do. I slightly blame America for my bodily obsession as it adds to my mental penetration. And of course, you blame your upbringing.

JOURNAL ENTRY 1999

My stomach HURTS. It always has to be all or nothing with me, so now I am stuck with all and an unhappy overdose of food in my body. I have decided that I want to marry, have a family and the whole nine yards. So I must lose weight, become a model size 2 (or maybe it's -2,) and then get some fabulous man to escort me down that long aisle to my dream life, where there are no cubicles or secretaries or any other aspects of corporate America. What I don't get is that many men run to Wall Street to make a shit load of money because they think this will land them a wife. Not all women associate marriage with money, but I guess a lot do. The irony in the whole mess is that most of those men that start on Wall Street to make that money to score that hot chick end up being too late because they work their asses off for several years in their twenties and early thirties and by the time they actually hit the bars or dating scene, the women have been scooped up by some other guy who said, "You got a great ass." Yup, that's all it took. Then, somehow, some Wall Street boys find time to squeeze women into the picture because there are 80-year-old women shopping on Madison as we speak with their 80-year-old Wall Street icon husbands sitting down in their corner office so there is some hope, I suppose, if you're okay with that sort of thing. So what if they have some putty-tang on the side. You turn away, just turn away. Hopeless.

JOURNAL ENTRY 1999

God, what has become of me? I can't even speak that name without wondering when I will have religion or faith in my life. Why do I think I need negative thoughts to drive me to greatness? Anger, bitterness, stubbornness. Such words seem to be valuable drivers to fame, fortune and personal physical fitness. Not love, compassion and peace. If you want to lose 10 pounds you don't think of happy thoughts, you take a picture of that one guy that rejected your sorry ass, and plaster it to the wall next to a naked ugly picture of yourself, and you use that every day to make you work out and drive you to a healthier happier self. So what if you use negative feelings to drive you, it doesn't make you a bad person, just the opposite, a better one. I just don't think that love can be the thing to save me these days, so it is out with the red and in with the black.

JOURNAL ENTRY 1999

I gave up reading Moby Dick today, because quite frankly, it sucks. I picked up D.H. Lawrence and read it in two days. Now, that's good writing. If you have to struggle to read it then it is probably quite bad.

It wasn't until ten years later that I realized why I liked D.H. Lawrence. There is a long list of bipolar writers that all paid homage to D.H. Lawrence.

Screams From the Balcony

By: Charles Bukowski

I have come through a green and red war these last 2 months. My side lost but I am still more alive than ever, in a sense. We have to pass through things, again, again – arguing with a knife blade, a bottle, weeping like a cunt in menopause, afraid to stop out a door...afraid of birds, fleas, mice...encircled by a clock, a typewriter, a half-open closet door full of ghosts, killers, horrors, like sea-bottoms. And then it ends. You are calm again. As calm as...a garage mechanic. I think of D. H. Lawrence title: Look We Have Come Through.

These were writers that also suffered from manic depression. Was it a coincidence that some paid homage to Lawrence? No. They loved him because he spoke to their brain because they had a similar brain. I continue to do research and realized that there is a longer list of writers that suffered from a mental illness, specifically bipolar disorder, who used the same diction, same syntax, and same stylistic techniques of similes and metaphors when they wrote. I can pick up a poem written by a bipolar writer and without knowing they were bipolar I could call it out, which means that you could track a mental illness simply by the way a writer puts words together. It was quite the discovery but not something a regular person would understand. How can you understand something that you don't have inside your own head?

JOURNAL ENTRY 1999

I spent my entire Sunday walking the street on Columbus and the Upper East Side, and stared at people, and watched them stare back at me. I am beginning to realize that we are not alone in our loneliness because everyone experiences the same loneliness. Some are just fortunate to enjoy spending time alone, and loathe the presence of others. I believe man is a creature of habit (I use the term man because it is a saying and stupid to change such catch phrases just to be politically correct). Thus, if he spends significant time alone, he is bound to get used to time alone, and not like to be with people. I am not one of those people. I have spent time alone, and still long to share it with familiar faces. But it is not the fifties, so I can't simply get wed to the first bachelor on the street. No, that would be way too simple and nice. Instead, I have to front a "career" for several years, earn a living and the respect of a mate, only to surrender it all to marriage. Well that makes a load of sense. Please let me work really hard to make a career, and meet men who respect my passion only to stop one day and stand in the kitchen, and watch the water run down the greasy pan while I hear the clock tick behind me three times. It's time to pick up the kids. Well that's not so bad, right?

JOURNAL ENTRY 1999

Ryan came up to Columbia for a funeral and actually called me to come see him. I went to his old frat house where everyone was hanging out, just like old times, but now there was the dark blanket of suicidal death coupled with murder. One of his friends on his sports team had lost it, decapitated his girlfriends head before jumping in front of a train and he was there to pick up the dusty pieces and toss it on his elevator going down grave. I ended up staying the night with Ryan and he actually cuddled with me.

Later the next day, after work, I met up with him and the group and flocked to an old bar on Amsterdam that I used to go to back in senior year. When we got there, I realized that Ryan had liquid acid on him and asked me if I wanted to try some. What the hell. Sure.

Go ahead and tilt my head back and drop it in my eye, where the blood vessels can soak it up fast and good. Faster than on the tough tongue where vessels sit somewhere deep in the mouth. Go straight to the soft source of the red frisbee rim holding my eyeball in place. I was down for just about anything, so got on board with the rest of the guys and drank some into my not blind eye. I was always after something more to push me farther and farther just to see how far I could go. I actually wanted a drug that put me to a place that released me from the ongoing impulse to challenge my brain. I suppose I wanted to match the excessiveness that my brain strived for. It was like a dare that I had to take up. There was nothing to put me over the edge and I don't know why I was constantly trying to get there. I lived on the edge. I ran toward the edge. The edge was all I knew. The edge was all I had. Once the acid hit, I was expecting something more, and was disappointed to find that it wasn't a big deal. My vision was askew, but that's about it. Next.

INVINCIBLE

Invincible
An insatiable appetite
Death never crosses the mind
Just more
Pushing the body like a rag doll
Because it can take it
The division of the mind from every limb
Makes it easy to think you can take more
Nothing in my mind stops the urge for more
When the body screams stop
You can't hear
The mind is all
And the body keeps going
Invincible
You think the body and mind share your being
When the mind wins every time
Telling you to have more
The pulses of the mind push human behavior
The body has no pull and the mind pushes forward
The ruler of your being
And the body keeps going
Now you can't stop
Your body stands alone in the struggle to share your space
But you've stopped listening
The brain is the size of your fist
And your muscles have no shot
In the war to listen
To your body
It's too late
The mind collapses and your body stops
Death becomes a word you know
Taught by the body
And excessive thoughts within the brain bring you to bed
The body wins.

"The Edge is What I Have"
By Theodore Roethke

Inside the Insane

What's madness but nobility to soul
At odds with circumstance? The day's on fire!
I know the purity of pure despair,
My shadow pinned against a sweating wall.
That place among the rocks – it is a cave,
Of winding path? The edge is what I have.

Canto III
By Lord Byron

Yet must I think less wildly: -I *have* thought
Too long and darkly, till my brain became
In its own eddy boiling and o'erwrought,
A whirling gulf of
Phantasy and flame:
And thus, untaught in youth my heart to tame,
My springs of life were poison'd.

Later that early morning, Ryan and I took a cab back to my place. It was finally going to happen and, of course, it was disastrous. I had my period and convinced myself that since it was toward the end, it wouldn't make an appearance. But of course, it did. Ryan freaked, jumped in the shower and got the fuck out of blood. I was left alone with the bright sunlight bolting through my windows. After four years of sitting in his smoky suite late nights again and again praying, thinking, after years of waiting there would be a time, he'll kiss you because you think he should, he must. And you fall asleep on his futon waiting for him to give in and let you sleep in his bed, because sitting near him is not enough but enough to keep you coming back with nothing to hold onto but the certainty that someday, one time, he'll give in, draw you in, hug you. After yearning for years it was over.

He went out the door and I didn't hear from him again. At least I didn't think I would...

CHAPTER 19

May 24, 2009 – CLOZARIL

For some patients stuck on the ward waiting for a bed, Ocean turns into a sun that beats down your sweat as you sit on an island stuck with the same surroundings, same people, same loneliness, same desperate attempt to get rescued, but there's only water around you. The ship that allows you to travel through life is nowhere to be found. You are stuck on the island of the insane.

Clozaril's future establishment, Sunny Side, called to let me know he might, might be going to the wondrous locked facility over the weekend. He had been taking Clozaril after much needed conversations about the necessity to take blood draws once a week. He didn't want to do it. But he wanted to stop seeing the three floating heads telling him to do things he could not avoid. I asked him what he preferred, floating heads or blood drawn from his arm once a week.

"I'd rather take the blood draws."

"Good. Because you need to do it. The Clozaril works." He nodded his head. He nodded it like he had to because he knew there was no other time or alternative that anything worked, despite his fierce attitude of 'I don't put needles in my blood and won't take it every week'. He was now. For now.

"It's like taking a vitamin. I get tired of popping vitamins every day but I do it. You don't get used to it but you do it because you have to." I thought about the truth. Yes, I did take a vitamin every morning, but I also had to toss back my own meds and so I knew the shitty frustration of knowing that you had to take meds and never knew if the day of not having to take anything would ever rise with the sun. Who was I kidding? Deep down and floating on the surface of the truth was that I knew I was going to have to take meds the rest of my life and that was that. He stood there with his weight medical flushed body growth and again nodded his head while rocking back and forth from left to right on his bare feet. He agreed to it. He took the blood draws and Sunny Side wanted to know what day he took them.

"Friday, he takes it today."

"OK." He took it that Friday, but not every Friday on the weekly schedule he was supposed to adhere to. But they made it be right enough to get him out. Get him to the next place. He was a 21-year-old kid with no family, no friends, who used to bum roaches off the street to get a tiny dismal hit of weed across his throat and was now going to Sunny Side. Well, ain't that something else. Ah...no.

June 1, 2009 – HOSPITAL HOPPING

Flaming Lips had a smear of lipstick on the right top lip of her angry tongue.
"I need cigarettes. Do you have any money?"
"No sorry, I don't." And I didn't. Why would I ever carry money on a ward that needed cigarettes, correction, money for cigarettes, more than coffee needs a mug.
"You can't get me cigarettes?"
"I want to talk to you about your discharge plan." She folded her hands like she had been down this business road before. And, we had been just a few weeks before.
"I can't go back to Apple Road?"
"Ah, no. You know I tried to get you back in there the first time and now we have to move to plan b."
"I want to go to a board and care."
"OK. Well I want to set you up with a HIH." She looked at me through her angry mouth and said nothing.

Two weeks later she was discharged to a board and care with an HIH. Three weeks later she was admitted to Eastside Memorial. They had a reputation of conserving patients. Flaming Lips was conserved. She was heading for Sunny Side, if they'd have her.

June 2, 2009 - BAM

Today an ecstasy junkie thrust a tiny Cambodian nurse's frontal lobe into a cement wall and ripped her hair out and was doing just fine before she tried to take his cheeseburger away from his thick hands. BAM. A less than quick beat and she was up against the wall like cement in between bricks and ready to suffer brain damage. She was not ready but no one was ready for any of this.

Skid Marks also lost it later that day. She was lonely, alone to the loneliest degree and couldn't take it anymore. Not that I am making excuses for her, but her level of care had changed so many times from locked to unlocked to locked to now what...? Top. I recalled from my initial conversation that she liked it there but one bad angry swipe to a staff member and a weekend in restraints, coupled with a potential personality disorder and fierce rejection from society and herself since brain fruition, now resulted in the highest level of locked facility out of all the locked down places in LA. One bad weekend and she kissed an open setting board and care good-bye. It was that flimsy. That random. Random behavior will screw you in a terrible way, but doesn't everyone suffer bad days?

June 3, 2009 – SUNSHINE

Sunshine. Sunshine wouldn't tell me why she spent four and a half months in jail. She had braids that stood out of her head like a palm tree.
"What's going on with your hair?"
"I'm making dreads."
"Oh."
"I was on the beach and I got beach lice."
"What's beach lice?"
"You know it lives in the sand. It jumps out when you move the sand and goes into your hair."
"That sounds gruesome. Jesus."
"Yeah."
"OK. Well I want to talk to you about a program called HIH." I went on to explain the program and she was so thankful for the opportunity to partake and have a support system out there that it gave me hope. So many HIH referrals connected the dots to steps to get wherever there was next. But connecting those dots was like being in kindergarten and trying to figure out which dots take that pencil to the next dot. It was a guess crap shoot coupled with pure luck. At least when you read those adventure books when you had a

choice to go from one adventure turning page to another you could go back and start over. Choose a different path, different page. You could even cheat and see what the ending was in the middle of the game. But not in real life.

The next day I had the HIH come and chat with her and she heard the word "shelter" and she was done. No thanks. The HIH tried to explain that a shelter was only an initial place to stay while they looked for another, better place. She wasn't having it. She came to LA from Florida for three weeks, which turned into over a year on the street and nowhere to go when she walked out the door. Which she did. Happily.

The HIH was then sent directly from that failed attempted to the 9th floor to interview another homeless person who had been on the streets for 20 years. He too heard the word shelter and backed out big time. I knew what the IMI's looked like, and sub acute care and enriched board and care living. And I knew that from the most needed help to the least needed help the conditions went from bad to real bad. I should have known the word shelter would freak someone out. It was at the bottom of the pool for help and it was the worse place possible. The worst place possible for people who needed a start, didn't need to be locked up at a facility, so once again, it was all ass backwards.

June 8, 2009 – BURNT

I took the day off. I'm definitely burned out. A year with no break breaks you. I woke up and didn't want to get out of bed, nevertheless, rolled out of bed, it was that bad. I'm in a major rut. And I'm in the field which means I more or less keep my own schedule. Until...

"Erica, I haven't seen you around very much." He was one of the attendings. I had not been to his rounds in about a month and at this point I didn't know how to get back to that 'I have to go to work' ethic. It was pretty bad. I hadn't talked with my open cases at all. Rotating Door was on the 9th floor and I would pass him in the hall. "I'll come talk to you tomorrow." I said it thinking that I would for sure, then didn't get my ass up there, or anywhere near the patients.

And it wasn't the patients that tired me, it was being on all the time. Being me, up, happy, open, a fresh breeze for the dealing staff that worked there. It was a lot of pressure to be on that level all the time. To be a relief.

"Hey, Loberg." And a satisfied that I was there smile would hit a face. I was tired. I was over me being me. I would be much better off chilling with the patients and talking to someone who was in and out and not expecting any production. Maybe that is what I have to do tomorrow to get my ass out of bed. The next week. Make it about the patients, only about the patients.

June 11, 2009 – KATRINA

Katrina was a 38-year-old black man. He was a survivor of Katrina and had moved quite a bit over the years. I sat down to talk with him about being his case manager and my heart fell. He had an athletic built, sad lips and big blood shot eyes. I explained that I could work with him to get him a place to stay without mentioning that there was a good chance the PG would conserve him and he would end up at Sunny Side. He was currently on a t-con, which was a temporary conservatorship for those patients that might be conserved, so I knew there was time to try and change that fate and get him a place like a board and care.

"Where did you stay before you were here?"

"A mission in Compton."

"Do you know what happened to lead you here?"

"I was writing on a chalk board and the police were out to get me." He went on to explain that he had been arrested over 40 times for minor things in his life. His current arrest was for entering a classroom at Compton College and writing on a chalkboard. He thought he was going to teach the students. After speaking with him for a bit I realized that he had been wandering around campus the majority of his life. He had a BA in accounting from Jackson College and enjoyed learning and an academic environment.

"Do you know what schizophrenia is?"

"Yes. I read about it in the library."

"Do you think you have it?"

"No." It was not a surprising answer, but I was surprised he had actually taken an interest in learning about something he didn't believe he had. As a Katrina survivor he migrated to Texas where apparently that was another cause for his arrest. He had said someone needed to kill Bush and just like that he was back in jail. However, given the terrible circumstances surrounding Katrina and Bush's handling of the situation, he sure didn't sound that insane to me. But when you are schizophrenic and speak your truth your ass is going to be on the line. Katrina agreed to work with me and I knew for some odd reason it was going to be a major challenge. I'm not sure if it was his sad eyes or his vagabond story, his broken relationship with his father, or his love for learning that always wound his ass back in jail. All he wanted to do was read in the library or teach a class and all the while he had schizophrenic mumblings that brought attention to him and made it impossible for him to be an academic.

June 18, 2009 – TB

I went to see Katrina today. I had been slightly dreading it because I knew his story, and not just his story but the way he walked, tall and necessary. It made me sad. I walked down the ward and peeped into his room and there was another person lying flat to his side on the bed. I was confused and briefly wondered if that meant he walked out the door, but knew he was temporarily conserved so he couldn't. Rounds started and I grabbed the current list of patients and there was an empty slot in the middle of the page, the slot that used to hold his name. I tried to concentrate on the doctors but couldn't take my fear of why he wasn't there, so got up and walked out. I went to the nurse's station and asked one of the nurses.
"Where's Katrina?"
"He's in seclusion on the med floor. His chest x-ray was positive for TB so they have him in seclusion." I'm not sure what my mind or heart felt at that moment. All I could do was envision this poor man lying all alone in a white room, afraid, and at the end of his end.
"Where is the med floor?"

Later that day I thought about the interview I conducted when opening his case and twice he excused himself to cough to the side. I knew TB traveled fast and far through the air and wondered what that meant for everyone else. I had already been exposed to TB a long time ago and was fortunate to be able to take an antibiotic for a year to ensure I would never get full blown TB. I would always be a carrier but never a victim. At least that's what I was told and now wondered if all the bent lies I told to the patients could come back to haunt me some day and leave me with some drowning lungs.

The next day I decided I would visit him. I knew he had no one and couldn't imagine how bad could turn to worse to even worse knowing that TB was in your chest and there was a bug in your brain and a fallen heart in your soul. I wandered to the med ER and they directed me to the med section of the hospital, but no one seemed to know where he was.

"I'm looking for a patient, Katrina W. He came in last night and is in seclusion for TB." Nurses kept redirecting me to another nursing station to another part of the dismal place and around and around I went with no answers to a final destination so I gave up. I didn't even know what the point was since I couldn't be near him anyway. Would he ever know if I was there? I knew he would never know that I tried, but I also knew he would probably return to the psych ward eventually.

A week later I found Katrina up on the 9th floor. They transferred him from isolation. I wondered if they moved him to the 9th floor because they didn't want to explain to everyone down on the 2nd floor why he had left and come back. No one seemed to know that he was admitted to the med floor for TB and no one wanted any red flag questions asked upon his return. I walked by his room a few times and he was always lying sideways facing the wall. I never saw him wander the halls or open his eyes. And I never made a move to see him face to face either.

June 20, 2009 – MORE ROTATING DOOR

I walked into Rotating Door's room to check in. He was busy reading the bible like most of the patients and I asked him his favorite section.

"Corinthians II and III."

"Why?" After I asked I was slightly sorry, for I knew his answer would be a long swirly whirlpool of ideas running here to there with very little page turning to hold it all together.

"Well, I'll come by and see you again tomorrow."

"What time?"

"Sometime in the afternoon."

"Like two?"

"Sure, sometime around then."

"OK." I remembered the last time I gave a specific time and it was for AWOL and he held me to it and was annoyed when I was twenty minutes late. I tried to keep the window loose because I never knew what my day would entail but I also knew that if it were me, I'd want a specific time so I could have something to structure my day or look forward to besides the candy cart lady who rolled down the halls a couple times a week or group time or a cigarette break, if you were actually well behaved enough to have one. As I was leaving I glanced over at the empty bed beside Rotating Door and there it was; the old rotted blood on the wall from the attack AWOL swore he endured. He had pointed to the blood to prove it and there it still was, a smear turned black with age beside the end of the bed. AWOL. No one believed him. And I still wondered, did that really happen? Wasn't the blood evidence enough?

CHAPTER 20

JOURNAL ENTRIES – MANHATTAN SPRING – 2000

Okay, I know I made a humongous mistake. Rule number one: Don't ever tell a boy you like him; it is the kiss of death. Number two: Never spend the night at his place on the first, second or third date, EVER! Now if only I could stick to one of the twenty goddamn rules, I just might land a mate. Just once, I want to meet someone that also doesn't play by the rules, but invents his own game. I deserve some honesty for once. I know there is something really bad inside of me, and I know this because it comes out sometimes. I curse a lot, and it bothers me, so I intend to really make an effort to stop. Wait...great! It's Lent very soon, and I have been looking for something to do that I can stick to. Why not no more dirty birdie language? Sounds great.

JOURNAL ENTRY

So now I am obsessed with a rock star, playing with a jockey, and have a few potential relationship in the works. Not too shabby...not too shabby. Now where is my future husband: London, New York, LA? Shit, what if he is NOT here but actually in Los Angeles or London? I'll tell you why I will never be alone, because I will always have writers and writers and more writers. Who needs companionship when you have two perfect eyes to read into the minds of thousands of writers: real people. Maybe they write fiction, but it stems from human experiences, right?

JOURNAL ENTRY

I don't do that well in the real world. My first "real job" out of college was working at a start up Internet company which blew out the door along with my ability to find another "real job", so now I have a temporary job. You work for random people in random jobs and most of the time you do absolutely nothing. I simply sit around and wait for someone to use my services and chill in a nice box and write. I write because my brain won't shut off. I recently read this book by Charles Bukowski. It was about this writer who had thousands of women of all types and ages; mostly hot young ones though. Anyway, he wrote about all his sex with various broads and they continued to enter his life because his writing about women somehow convinced them that he knew or understood women when he was really a filthy old man. The book is even called "Women." So maybe if I ever publish this shit some male will read and understand my voice, and my brain, and come find me. Great, this is my greatest newest plan ever.

JOURNAL ENTRY

I think people mostly write because they either have something to share, or nothing to do. Boredom can lead to writing. Yeah, boredom and meaninglessness definitely instigate the writing process. At least they do for me. But that means that what I write must be boring. Let me think of something interesting. I wonder when or if I am going to hit rock bottom. Can there be any way to stop the loneliness that consumes my soul? I must be lying on the rock bottom abyss all the time so, really, there will never be a rock bottom. I will always go to extremes, up, down, up, down, and there really is nothing I can do about it.

JOURNAL ENTRY

I never liked the phone and recently I've had a slight panic attack when I come home to a red light blinking on my answering machine. I don't want to check the messages. Checking means calling someone back which is too much effort right now.

JOURNAL ENTRY

I think my hyper nights stem from a deep depression. I am so lonely and tired that I can't deal. The depression takes hold and I am out on the town lashing out at society. I can only thank the angels that surround me and protect the people that cross my face.

JOURNAL ENTRY

I decided today I needed to get out of the dirty cement so I jumped on a train and headed north to visit my little sister Olivia at Yale for the weekend and…okay, so I am a serious pedophile, (technically I am not, but he was close enough to being underage that I can say I was a pseudo pedophile). However, if men can roam the earth and hit on women half their age AND get away with it, then why shouldn't I do the same!? Well, I did, as a matter of fact. I went a little bit crazy and yes, I macked on a freshman and I LIKED IT!! Okay, let's rewind. I arrived in New Haven on Saturday around noon, and got Olivia caught up on my life, its present, and its soon to be future. We pre-partied and I met my main squeeze early on in the night. Yaley. What a great lover, kisser, caresser, would be perfect make-out boyfriend and nothing else probably. We started our mack fest in the dirty grimy club-like bar in New Haven, and kept making out till 6:00 that next morning in his dorm room bed. Yes, his roommate was asleep on the top bunk, but I didn't care. The next morning I ended up casually saying goodbye even though there was a distinct sexual tension from outer space simmering down between us. How do you explain that? We'll just chalk it up to a notch for there is no future with some Yale frosh…so that is that….I suppose.

JOURNAL ENTRY

Okay, sometimes you need some good old hard honesty in your life. I am a man eater. I cannot get enough of boys, or the idea of them, if that is possible. Why are the last few sentences ending with such uncertain phrases like "I suppose" or "I guess"? I freaking know what I know and that is that!!!! I know my shortcomings, and long comings, and that I will always be obsessed with boys boys and more boys. Their hands, ass, hair, eyes, mouth, lips, stomach, legs, shoulders, hips, ass, (I already said that), their eyelashes. I just want to experience all of them, and not stop till I get enough. I can drink them up like a martini and still be hungry for more. I think everyone is born with an amount of passion, sexual desire and testosterone or estrogen and whatever that make-up is that determines your ability to obsess about boys and need them. For example, some people get hungry five times a day while others only get hungry once or twice a day. Some people have a high metabolism and others have a low one, so when it comes to the hunger of sex, my body requires more then the average Cinderella. I am not talking about just sex, but love and passion. There is a difference between sexual drive, and passionate drive. Passionate drive is one's ability to thirst for love and a soft touch to caress your body. I can sit and kiss with a good kisser for hours and still not get enough. My body would still need more, more and more. Some people need to drink from the river of love more than others, so should we be docked for that? No. We should just dock our boat on that stream. But someone should explain the reasoning for this and appease all those poor souls that think they are weird for having a particular capacity for passion. I just don't want to get hurt, which means I always have to keep my gold to myself. I will only dish over my gold once I am walking down that aisle. Once, when….the scariest word in the world: IF.

Passion is a live killer in the soul because it screams inside your seams and no one else gets it. Passion can appear as crazy or wild or too hardcore. Why is a burning fire in the heart a bad thing? I suppose if you lack passion then standing by an open flame seems scary. We fear what we don't understand. When we have no barometer to test the land of internal combustion then it can all come off as odd. When people don't have different chemicals fueling their passion, it's hard to understand the enthusiasm of an alive being. A human alive being sizzling in the middle of the flame.

I think now is a good time to admit that I have an abnormal amount of sexual drive to the point where I am wild. A hypersexual being that would masturbate ten times a day if there were places in public that I could go do that.

JOURNAL ENTRY

I thought about Ryan today. God, what a disaster it was the last time we saw each other when he was in town for his friend's suicide funeral. And to think his friend was in one of my classes sophomore year. It's interesting how I never have suicidal thoughts yet, when I am flying around town, I act suicidal. I have no control over myself but definitely think that I do, when really I am this wild soul acting outside of myself. Well, it is myself, but it's an extension of myself that is so out of hand that I am slightly shocked that I am still here.

HER KIND
By Anne Sexton

I have gone out, a possessed witch,
haunting the black air, braver at night;
dreaming evil, I have done my hitch
over the plain houses, light by light:
lonely thing, twelve-fingered, out of mind.
A woman like that is not a woman, quite.

I have been her kind.

I FORGET WHAT IT'S LIKE 2010

I forget what it's like
To scream in the streets
Sheltering a scramble
Because I know
To hold
Myself in.

When I'm throwing myself
Out
Into the night
Like a person
Walking up to your dinner table
Sitting down
And starting a conversation
With you
And your party
Hi how are you doing
Or
How's that salad
I've had it, it's OK.

It's surprising to recall those tossed up honest
Thrusting nights
In and out of here
And that place
And then let's go there

And all the time
Beside the internal furiousness
The steps keep stride
Of block
Enough
To keep you physically
In line
And you're in line
Inside your brain
Because you know what it's like
Yourself that well
That when you are scrambling across the streets
Like a parachute on your heels that you can still take charge
And keep your skin in place
Because internally your brain jumps so hard against the thick
knowing voice of
You are in control
That you maintain control.
You get accustomed to it.
Or else…

There is no or else. It's you.

JOURNAL ENTRY

My younger sister Olivia came to visit me today. She is the only person in my life who I can actually depend on. She is the only person who I can talk to. She is probably the spirit that keeps me from going over the edge. She was kind enough to take a train from New Haven to visit me. She walked into my apartment and surveyed the place. It was the first time she'd seen my new pad on 77th. Well, it's more of a white walled square mothball, but it was mine.

"Wow!"

"What?" I was getting ready to go out and applying my usual mascara mixed with brown eye shadow.

"What are all these?" She was observing my wall of cards and was slightly perturbed.

"It's my stable."

"There are so many." I had the feeling she was trying to hide the

shock wave most likely penetrating throughout her body while she looked at the wall of cards. I didn't think it was a big deal.
"I have a system. See, the first column are guys I just met that I am dating. The next are guys I've gone on a few dates with but are being phased out. And the last column are guys I am not sure I will ever hear from or talk to again so they get rotated out as new cards pour in." It all seemed very logical to me. We went out that night and I managed to collect a few more cards to add to the wall.

JOURNAL ENTRY

So I am left with a huge query: Do I move to LA? I am so confused and feel like such a failure at this point. God, I went through so many men this year. So many dates and disappointments left and right. Enough already. I am tired of always making the effort and hitting on random men. Let them come to me for a change. Maybe my luck will change in the land of the lost and stupid. Maybe I will be the first writer ever to write a positive novel about LA. A writer demands a difficult capacity: a serious brain, and an acute awareness of the human spirit. I have some of both but more of the former I think. We shall see.

JOURNAL ENTRY

The past year of my life I have been in a very dark place, and it keeps getting darker. I don't know why I have been in such a dark place this past year. I feel like my body has been through some war of some sort and I am only 22 years old. I need to remember it is a sacred temple and take better care of the inside.

Maybe it was the rejection I never felt but bottled up that made me lash out all year. When Carter rejected me, I never let myself feel it, or admit it, so it left me suppressing that void that everyone carries around. Some are lucky. Some fill the void with positive things like people, love, spouses, family and friends. I chose to avoid the reality of that void and fill it with random men I happened to meet on the street, in the bar, on the bus, you name it, I met it. It is no way to be or live, and I am happy that I can finally see the sun. Since I am blessed with obsessive-compulsive disorder, I think, I might as well utilize its force to make it right. Tired. It's Friday. I wonder how I go out and stay up till five in the morning and am not tired the next day. Am I fooling myself? Am I going to all of a sudden hit a wall of exhaustion and want to die?

I fear the clock.

CHAPTER 21

June 23, 2009 – SKIDDED OUT

Skid Marks left for Top today. She went from an IMI to a board and care to an enriched board and care to a referral to a sub acute and was now at the top of the crazy chain at Top state hospital. I felt OK about it though. She wanted it. At least that day we spoke about it. And all was quiet on the Ocean ward front. Skid Marks's moaning and groaning and constant call to "Get me out of here" had finally ceased. She was gone and the unit was quiet. For now.

June 26, 2009 – THE CUTTER

We had a cutter in rounds today. She was a young 98-pound 20-year-old girl who didn't like to be alone. She had been on Zoloft recently and increased the dosage which supposedly could cause a reverse effect and lead to depression. Her cuts weren't that bad and the doctor was having a hard time getting any answers.
"Why did you cut yourself?" She sat with a stoic stare and her toes jumped up and down under the table.
"What did you use?"
"Scissors."
"What kind of scissors?"
"Child's scissors." The doctor wasn't getting too far and her tears slowly streamed down her face beneath her glasses. After a few more questions she was released. We went back to talking about patients and there was a man who only liked blue and white and so would only take blue or white meds and the table went through a gamut of different pills trying to decide which ones were blue or white for him to take. X med, X med, X med...the list went on and on and I wondered how it was possible to actually run through so many potential pills for a patient to pop. The method had zero accuracy but neither did his diagnosis of schizophrenia NOS. Not Otherwise Specified. Everything always had a NOS piggy backed onto it. The patient's charts also had over five different diagnoses in

it. No one seemed to have a clear understanding of what the patient had, so would just write what was convenient at the time. That was why so many had PDNOS. Then half way through the chart there would be another diagnosis, then another, then..hell, what did it matter. The diagnosis changed as often as the meds and every patient seemed to have at least two different mental diseases.

Toward the end of rounds the doctor mentioned his problem with the parallels between creative genius and mental illness. He thought the meandering mind of a bipolar individual release coupled with the inability to complete a task made the argument for a correlation between creative genius and bipolar or schizophrenia unlikely. This argument had been an ongoing emphasis that seemed to get under his skin as it was an argument on a wide spectrum of understanding mental health. Not to mention the other argument about medication playing a role in stifling the creative thought process. He did make one concession and commented.

"Maybe with one exception: bipolar II. A hypomanic state may produce creative thought during an episode. And with lithium it could slow down that process. But hypomania would be the only one close to standing on two legs for an argument for a relationship to creative genius." I thought about my writing process, how I would have to jump out of bed in the middle of the night when there was something I had to write about. I would go for runs and run over my writings in my head and would have to race home to capture it, or release it. Release the possession that writing had over my mind, my soul, and by being. No one chooses to be a writer, writing chooses them. Sometimes it felt like a curse cause I didn't have a choice. I had to do it. My thoughts would skyrocket out of my brain in a Niagara Falls crush and pen itself onto the page. It wasn't till years of tampering with all forms of writing that I found a medium that worked. Poetry. Poetry was easy cause it was short and sweet. I could observe something or feel something and could pull out my back pocket memo pad and write it down. On the train, at a park, walking down the street, there was material everywhere that my mind sucked in and I could have a moment of relief when I got it out of my brain and onto the page. But the relief after the release of thoughts communicated on the page only lasted till the next possession took hold. And I never knew when it would happen. Was it a demon or a friend? I guess it doesn't matter cause it wasn't in my hands. Walking into a patients room peeled my eye to creative thoughts that required constant appeasing as I banged down the doors of my head to let it live. Tell the truth in what your mind sees, what it feels, and always keep it real. Give it all or leave your mind to hell. The problem was I never had time to think. I couldn't control the speed of my mind and it flew through the ink of my pen without any breath. Write write write or die inside your mind of fluid thoughts that refused to shut down. My poetry seemed to be the only medium I could trust cause it mirrored the beats of my brain unlike any other form of writing. And it was convenient. I could write a poem and it was done. A mere moment of observation came to life in a poetic party that I never had to clean up. I never went back to rewrite or rethink my thoughts that I was fortunate to get down then and there. When my heart was crushed and I felt the pain of love or loss in emotional tears I couldn't go back and find that moment of intense feelings. I couldn't retear so when it was captured and released it was done. Over. No editing, no rereading. Next. My mind would never rest and that was a fact I was able to temper with my poetry. Poetry was easy. Easy to write, and it was easier not to have the bible of other writings hang over my head. I wouldn't have to go back to the pages upon pages of writings over the last decade and try to edit it or put it together into one coherent piece. The sheer beauty of poetry is it could represent my mind in punctuation, capitalization, swift beats flavored with random metaphors and the juxtaposition of words that may not seem right, but it was how my brain saw things and somehow provided a template for how my brain functioned. Screw *The Elements of Style* by Strunk and White. Poetry had no rules and I swam in love in it. When your mind screams and you tack on exclamation points back to back until the scream subsides you learn about the mechanics of your mind. My mind saw things so detailed that every word counted and had a place. Maybe having a twisted mind that saw the lead in the tip of a pencil instead of the whole pistol made it hard to be understood in the world, but the trade off, getting excited over words and how they worked together side by side and up and down from line to line on a page, was worth it. And I was not alone. It wasn't until I read other manic writers that I saw parallels in their writings and was able to find friends in their work. The excitement of their minds in words bursting on the page allowed me to see inside their being. Samuel Taylor Coleridge was my friend. The icon of a hypomanic poet that proved poetry was a craft suitable for a hypomanic person and it showed how a chemical imbalance in the brain can be read in the words on a page. And as a hypomanic individual I wasn't going to suffocate my mind which left me no choice. I had to write. And poetry chased me.

Excerpts from "Biographia Literaria"
By Samuel Taylor Coleridge 1817

During the first year that Mr. Wordsworth and I were neighbors our conversations turned frequently on the two cardinal points of poetry--the power of exciting the sympathy of the reader by a faithful adherence to the truth of Nature, and the power of giving the interest of novelty by the modifying colors of imagination. The sudden charm which accidents of light and shade, moonlight or sunset, diffuse over a familiar landscape appeared to represent the practicability of combining both. ("What is a Poem?)

At school I had the advantage of a very sensible though severe master. I learned from him that poetry, even that of the loftiest odes, had a logic of its own as severe as that of science, and more difficult, because more subtle. In the truly great poets, he would say, there is a reason assignable, not only for every word, but for the position of every word. ("The Nature of Poetic Diction")

THE JUXTAPOSITION OF WORDS 2005

Words go together

Across a page

Zippingly spicy

Warm and softly tired and slow

Ready and bleeding

Boringly blind.

The juxtaposition of words.

Metaphors

Plopping of ideas

In a sentence

It's not random

It tells the mind

In its purest form.

June 28, 2009 – SURE, CALL 911

The 2nd floor is doing interviews now during rounds. The residents must have complained. Some tended to bitch and whine like the old stereotype of entitlement that goes along with always introducing someone as "Doctor" so and so. We interviewed a young 22-year-old guy who had problems sleeping. And that was when things started to unwind inside me.

"There is no number to call when you can't sleep" he said. It made sense to me.

"911 is the number you call." The doctor said it like maple in syrup. Like oh right, like THAT is the obvious answer. You can't sleep so call an ambulance. Ridiculous. Call 911? If I called 911 from ages 5 – 28 every time I couldn't sleep...I don't even have an end to that sentence, it is that ridiculous. Call 911. Okkkay.

Erica Loberg

INSOMNIA

How do you explain how the eyes burn?

If I had a gun I'd shoot the birds
Sleep is an old habit
So old you forget.

What it's like to feel your eyes simmer.

You close the steady balls of cotton
Dipped in alcohol
Smiling open inside
Awake
Behind the lids
Stinging more than before.

You are the dead
And alive in the burn.

Like the wood of a bonfire
Almost asleep on the beach
The orange logs get slowly cooked to death

While the sun rises.

Your burn remains.

JOURNAL ENTRY – MANHATTAN - 2000

I haven't slept more than a few hours this past week and my
eyeballs burn. I feel like there is a wheel turning inside me and it
runs so fast that I could win a Nascar race. Time is so slow I want to
shoot myself. I feel like an hour should be ten and it drives me up a
wall onto the ceiling and back down again.

CHAPTER 22

August 4, 2009 – AWOL RETURNS

AWOL is back. One of the social workers got a phone call from Eastside Memorial and he was in their psych ward. Apparently he had awoled from LA transportation on his way to the courthouse for a hearing. I imagined his agile self bursting away from the van and escaping the scene. He did have a hefty track record for awoling. I recalled his enthusiastic borderline hysterical interpretation of his awol from Shoreline. He was really into it and probably was able to use that same innate energy to bust out of dodge yet another time. It didn't last long though. He did something to bring his ass back to the psych ER. What that was, I didn't know, nor did I want to.

August 6, 2009 – ROTATED OUT

Rotating Door left today. I didn't want to go say goodbye but thought the wounds of my sad goodbye to Preggers were finally healed. Actually, I more or less felt guilty for not working more with Rotating Door and it was apparent when we crossed each other in the hall.

"Rotating Door. You're going today." I was as upbeat as possible and held my breath, hoping that he knew he was going and where he was going.

"Yeah." His eyes were solemn and his stomach protruded out on the catwalk. He had gained a significant amount of weight since his arrival a few months ago and it showed. Not that he cared.

"Well that's exciting."

"Where have you been? I haven't seen you around."

"I've been on the 2nd floor. You remember the 2nd floor? The dungeon?"

"Yeah."

"I don't want to see you back here. OK?"

"OK." I turned with my key to the door to my office in hand and he put his hand out. I shook his hand and the door was ajar. Before I stepped across the threshold I stopped myself and turned to face him. He stood there alone.

"I'll pray for you." The look on his face said that it truly meant something to him.

"Thank you." I smiled goodbye and disappeared into the hallway. As I walked out the doors later that day I thought about the weight of the words I will pray for you to someone who lived by the bible every day and every meal. I couldn't recall the last time I actually prayed and hoped that I would remember to pray for him that night. At least once was enough for me to get by without feeling like I should have done more.

August 7, 2009 – JUST SAY IT ALREADY

I got the call today.

"Hey, Erica. I wanted to talk to you about coverage." I knew it was coming. I also knew the topic would be broached in that particular manner.

"Nicaragua's last day is next Wednesday and we have hired a person to replace her but she doesn't have a start date yet." Of course she doesn't. I managed to get a kind of lie answer out of her regarding the duration of this "coverage."

"Ah..it could be a few weeks or months. You know how the county is." I still didn't understand what that meant. She thanked me for agreeing to do it and I wanted to hang up with the truth: I didn't really have a choice in the matter. I didn't say it then but did later in person the next time I was in the office. The list of county requests were piling onto my tired car. We are billing for the county so open up cases...we need you to cover two hospitals till the other person starts...whenever that would happen. Would the open cases pressure cease once the county had more money...? It's interesting to see what uncovers itself in times of crisis. I'm spread thin driving from Ocean to Eastside and backed up against the wall to open cases because...it's for the patients. OK. Got it.

August 26, 2009 - EASTSIDE

I'm at Eastside Memorial and it's nice. It's nice in the way that is

not Ocean. People are open. Not hard.
"Hi, my name is X. It's nice to meet you. Let me show you the nurse's station" type of thing. There is not hierarchy or deflation of spirit but isolated honesty. They work in their cells and make progress happen.

I have officially crossed the dirty tiles. But at Eastside the tiles weren't dirty. The halls were quiet and the place was clean. It must be Santiago that made the place so unlike the old shit on grimy heels that rested in between my hair at Ocean. Santiago roamed the halls with his trashcan licking the place clean with his plastic bags and Mexican smile. It was a new place. A fresh start inside an old habit. Eastside Memorial is now my official home, for now. Treatment is different here, as are the patients. They don't seem to be over-medicated or have outrageous outbursts which is really a contradiction, because if you are over-medicated you don't have rage episodes and if you are under-medicated maybe you do; I don't know. Again, I am not a doctor, but am now thrown into a whole new work environment with different attendings and nursing staff and social workers and medical caseworkers. I don't miss Ocean. I miss some of the people there, but not all the drama. In the end The Demon's constant shit in my face got the best of me. She managed to wheedle me out of most social work responsibilities so I really didn't see a point in being there. The Demon couldn't stand the fact that most of the patients wanted to work with me more than her coveted social work staff. It drove her up the wall, so she drove me into the ground. It was sad because I liked so many of the people there, but I knew it was time for change. It was past time for change. My replacement is definitely not happy there and does not feel welcome, so all my efforts to set up a more comfortable position for the new coming liaison was pointless. People don't change and the system remains the same. Eastside Memorial doesn't seem to discharge people as much and leans toward conservatorship. I am not so hot on conservatorship so find it a hard adjustment, but maybe it has its benefits. They do keep their patients here longer for treatment which is good, but locking them up when they are a borderline case is not. They are very wary of discharging people to "the street", for it is a sensitive topic that can be front page news. But there were ways to work around the discharge to self plan as long as nobody says those scary words "to the street." It reminded me of the time one of the residents in rounds at Ocean said the patients were "snowed" due to too many meds.

"We don't use that term here." Snapped back in his face. Maybe there's a better way to describe it: caught in an avalanche of face packing snow?! Or a dust whirlwind in the desert? I had a quick flashback of one of my patients on the 9th floor.

THE WALRUS

The Walrus
Sits across from me
So heavily medicated
That he can't put letter
After letter
To form a word
Together.

Eyes and lips barely open
"Same Day Paint and Body"
Sweatshirt
With dribble
Down the front
Hardened by days
Possibly weeks
Of continual wear
But no tear.

JOURNAL ENTRY – BANK BLVD. - 2006

"What do you think about Bank Blvd.?"
"Ha, your funny." Carter moved to LA and was living on the street I grew up on. By happenstance. After more years than dirty tears put together on the bleak ward.
"I grew up on Bank." I'm sure he could hear my face over the phone.
"Oh." Like it didn't matter. Okayyyyy.
"What are you doing later?"
"Ah, I don't know." Carter didn't know me. He didn't know that I never made plans. It's not like I had commitment issues. I just had issues period. I never knew what I was doing the next week, the next day, that day, it was all what I felt like right before I sat down to read. Always.
"You want to come over and watch TV?"
"Sure."
"OK, see you later."
"Bye."

We reconnected. We picked up where our friendship was freshman and sophomore year. Friends that hung out like branches on a tree. We ignored the years that past and spent every friendly night hanging out together and we were back where we always seemed to be. Just friends, but not really. I was still convinced that deep down he liked me. Deep down he had Pandora's box and it was closed but it was there nonetheless. I didn't know if he liked me but wouldn't admit it to himself, or liked me and didn't know that he did. Either way it sucked. And I didn't even get to use my skills to help change his mind an eighth way around to hopefully get it screwed on right. Either way I was not going to be his girlfriend. We had sex randomly a couple times which made no sense, but nothing about our relationship ever made sense. Spending every night together and talking for hours on his balcony didn't make even more sense. And telling him about my mental problems didn't seem like the right thing to do, just yet, till eventually I did. I had to because he saw me more and more every day and hiding needing help wasn't an option at the time.

Then he introduced me to Dean.

CHAPTER 23

October 15, 2009 - THE STAGE

Her name was The Stage. She was a tiny woman in her late fifties with tired gray uncombed hair with a sideways bow stuck to the side of her head. It was too late to file for conservatorship and she didn't want to go home to her husband because he was the "Queen of Spain." She went on voluntary stay and the $ 2,400 a night stay had to come to an end. The plan was simple. Get her out of the door, off county property, a simple step on the cement sideway, and the ambulance team could come and pick her up and bring her back so she could finally be conserved and spend the rest of her life at Shoreline. She only liked one person on the ward and she was a sweet old nurse. The Stage was determined to go home with her.

"I'm going home with the nurse" she would say day after day, as she refused to acknowledge her husband. The nurse was set to be the bait to her outside.

"Come on The Stage. We are going to go now." She thought she was going home with the nurse as she stepped outside the hospital doors and meandered onto the sidewalk. The one problem was, she had to do something to be brought back onto the ward and that something was yet to be determined. Everyone watched as she stood outside beside the nurse waiting for her car. No car appeared and she began to walk down the street.

"God, this is so sad." I mumbled outside of my breath.

"Why? We are helping her." The social worker believed in the cause.

"By staging a 'you're going home with the only person you trust' when really you are going back to the slammer? On what charge are they going to bring her back?"

"She is gravely disabled. Look, she is confused and wandering down the street." She was confused but she wasn't harming herself or anyone and it was a hell Mary call to say she was "gravely disabled." But the ambulance was already called and the PMRT (Psychiatric Mobile Response Team) to take her back in had already been aware of the plan so were waiting patiently. And she stood there. Waiting for the nurse's car. Waiting to go home when the ambulance pulled up. I couldn't bear to see her reaction to the restraints. Her reaction to the surprise attack and gurney wheels that would wheel her back to her room. To her hospital second home. She was now on my radar for placement. She would get conserved and end up at Shoreline. The whole thing was a show. I'm surprised they didn't hand out a script to make sure everyone knew their lines, their scenes and their role in leading this lady home. Home would be Shoreline. Shoreline was the shittiest place in all of the IMI's. But, on a fresh breath note, Eastside had a different philosophy and methodology for treating and discharging patients. They didn't over-medicate people to calm their bones long enough to get them green lit discharged...wherever. They challenged a system that demanded patients be rotated out like a pez dispenser. They did their best to make a plan that worked for the individual in a county that ran on a different set of stretcher wheels. The county demanded that hospitals move people out at an accelerated pace, so what can you do? Jab pills down a patient's throat to temporarily suffocate their disease till they get released? That's an option that seemed to take center stage at Ocean. So who is to blame? Finger pointing is a waste of time cause it's a dusty bag full of tricks, however, the first finger pointer should go ahead and stick their thumb up their ass cause it only underscores an insecurity that you may just be part of the problem.

I later took the elevator with the nurse and saw the old tears holding ground inside her eyes. She was the star of the show and she played her part beautifully but I knew she didn't like the movie. She didn't like the deception and would have to carry that home. To her home alone with no The Stage by her side.

November 2, 2009 – TIME TO GET THE FUCK OUT OF A FUCKLESS TOWN

It was time to leave boy's town aka West Hollywood. The commute was getting to be too much. It wasn't until I moved to Downtown LA that I realized that I had wasted a lot of my twenties living in the wrong environment. Boy's town was just that, strictly for boys.

I moved. I walked the streets and found my loft. It was a fresh breath of petals up my nose. Downtown living is all I have to say. Downtown living. And I loved it.

December 5, 2009 – AGITATED VS. IRRITABLE

The patients have one word that is the dart to their locked cell. Agitated. It was a common word scrawled across the chart that kept all the patients dirty outside secrets inside. If you were agitated you oftentimes needed a time out. Is there a fine line between irritability and agitation? Possibly. But that line is thickly fine enough to make a difference. Agitation in a bipolar I person can stick on the sleeve for awhile and irritability comes at a bipolar II split moment when you drop your shoe and they are not sitting left and right by each other and there is a quick shock of irritability inside the skin that comes out of nowhere and then it's gone.

Yes, when I was a younger than young I tore off some shutters. Yes, I threw a few quick comets in the sky attacks here and there at my sister. By accident. I couldn't control my emotions tearing out physically all over some of the air in front of my family's faces, arms, hair. Or my bursting tears. Telling me over and over that I'm too sensitive is like saying you have too many freckles. Hyper sensitivity, hyper emotional, hyper energetic. Hyper is a pre word to a word that for everyone else is normal. There is no such thing as "hyper" anything when in your world that is normal. I couldn't control it. I can try and stay out of the sun but it'll find me. How do you make someone understand you're sorry when your irritability happens so fast that you don't realize you've done something till after the blood, the tears, the look of what the fuckkkk!?

"Alone"
By Edgar Allan Poe

From childhood's hour I have not been
As others were—I have not seen
As others saw—I could not bring
My passions from a common spring—
From the same source I have not taken
My sorrow—I could not awaken

Erica Loberg

My heart to joy at the same tone—
And all I lov'd—I lov'd alone—
Then—in my childhood—in the dawn
Of a most stormy life—was drawn
From ev'ry depth of good and ill
The mystery which binds me still—
From the torrent, or the fountain—
From the red cliff of the mountain—
From the sun that 'round me roll'd
In its autumn tint of gold—
From the lightning in the sky
As it pass'd me flying by—
From the thunder, and the storm—
And the cloud that took the form
(When the rest of Heaven was blue)
Of a demon in my view—

CHAPTER 24

JOURNAL ENTRY - MANHATTAN IRRITABLE VS.
AGITATED - 2000

Okay, so I am feeling better about the extent to which I am taking advantage of the temping experience to write my words of madness because I have come to realize that the people who I work for also know the beauty of the temping system. They don't pay for my services, and do you think some big ass CEO of some gigantic company knows where every nook and cranny hides in an entire Thomas English Muffin? Okay, so the Human Body Experience is reducing me to food metaphors, but that is all I have left these days. It's a new project. It is called "The Human Body Experience." The HBE is an experiment I have decided to undergo. I plan on not eating until my birthday, which is one and a half months away. During that time, I plan to lose 15-20 pounds of real fat. Fat that has been on my body my entire life and has plagued me. I sit on the toilet, look down, and there it was every time without fail. A roll of lard with a smiling crease above it mocking me. I would lie in the bathtub and it was there, weighing me down in the water. I wanted out, and I had to go to the utmost extreme to get it. I even managed to cut out frozen yogurt, which I thought would NEVER occur in this lifetime. Anyway, so the CEO decides to downsize because the word on the street in major companies is it's the thing to do so they add a few temps here and there to accommodate this loss. And why not? A temp requires no benefits or commitment, so why not take a few to make up for the hundred stems you fired this month? But in actuality, there is no need for that much extra help so the people on the lower tiers work the temping system to the max. They have their little call girl to perform miscellaneous tasks and aren't surprised when the temp appears busy because, well, anyone can call on you at any time to do some bullshit.

When I needed a break from the bullshit I would hit up the Au Bon Café at the bottom of my building. If you are going to pay serious gold for some java make sure it is done properly!!! I ordered a cappuccino, and first got some sort of coffee with some milk splashed on the top and took it back and asked for some more foam

Erica Loberg

and got another of the same sorry cross between a café au lait and a latte but decided I didn't need a fight today because I woke up feeling dizzy to begin with and needed some juice to kill the bird fluttering around my brain. So I walked over to the accessories stand and was ready to dress my juice and turn it into a JOLT! Twenty packets of Equal can do the trick, and two, not three jabs of cinnamon (three causes the cinnamon to sink to the bottom and melt into a syrup substance that can be quite disgusting if you happen to gulp it down on your last sip and usually I did) and I was off. Walking to the elevator I took a sip...COLD!!!!!! Okay I am exaggerating, but it was definitely lukewarm and not up to my $3.10 standards. I marched back into the store and walked to the register.

"Hi. I ordered a cappuccino with skim milk and it is warm."
"I can't help you. Go ask them down there." He motioned to the end of the bar, and I dreaded having to go back to the same dolt for a third attempt at some love.
"Yes, I know I should go down there but this is my second coffee from your colleague over there so do you think you can find someone who can make me a cappuccino the right way please?" I was trying my best to be pleasant, but who can be pleasant on a Tuesday morning after fifteen minutes of coffee shop hell?
"I am sorry. Our manager is over there." I didn't want to speak to the manager, and one look at this so called manager made me realize I had no hope in finding some peace in a hot shot of dirt drenched in fake sugar and spruced up milk with a dollop of brown coating.
"Fine!" New boy to the rescue. A new coffee maker was busy making coffee while the F- was handling the bagel bar. The new boy handed me the drink.
"Is this with skimmed milk? Sorry, I am lactose intolerant." Not a total lie, but I needed to watch the Human Body Experience and I knew I would break it later with some Canterbury chocolate eggs I would steal from the cubicle next to me, so every ounce of fat at this point counted. He took it back to make again and the bagel boy was making it everyone's business to know I was a high maintenance loudmouth coffee snob who should take my package and leave. I was not moving and chanted in my head "the customer is always right...the customer is always right." And I was. I received the blessing and walked back to the table and redid my previous ritual and finally had my juice. I could never go back. Not because I am

ashamed of my actions, but think the service sucks and doesn't deserve my gold. I obviously have some irritability issues, but doesn't everyone?

Ok. So I came across as a total asshole. My irritability got the best of me most of the time in that period of my life. However, to see my actions and the term "irritability" used to describe my mental state ten years ago, speaks to my belief that mental illness can be discovered through the content in writings. Stylistic techniques also share a component in understanding and discovering mental illness. All capitalizations followed by exclamation points can be a window into the mind of a passionate or irritable person. When I was on a manic high my writing would change. The words would shoot off the page and punctuation manifested my brain in a particular state of mind.

So I walked over to the accessories stand and was ready to dress my juice and turn it into a *JOLT!*
Walking to the elevator I took a sip...*COLD!!!!!!*

Did I really need six explanation points to make my point? No. But my mind had to, because that's what it felt at that irritable moment and that's how it expressed itself. I was in a manic irritable state and the diction described it.

"They shut me up in Prose."
By Emily Dickinson

Still! Could themself have peeped --
And seen my Brain -- go round --
They might as wise have lodged a Bird
For Treason -- in the Pound –

"Portions of a Wine-Stained Notebook"
By Charles Bukowski
"Death batters at my mind like a wild bat enclosed in my skull"

"I woke up feeling dizzy to begin with and needed some juice to kill the bird fluttering around my brain."
By Erica Loberg

If I had known then that irritability beyond a reasonable shrink and the image of a bird or a bat fluttering around the mind to describe the inner working of the brain could possibly be a sign of a mood disorder, things would have been very different the last ten years.

CHAPTER 25

January 1, 2010 – THE CANNON BALL, LITERALLY

My cat fell out of the window today. Or at least I think it was today, or sometime last night. I'm not sure. I came home and he was gone. I searched in places that you would rarely find a squeezed cat stuffed into and it hit me like cold rain down your back. He is gone. The doorman told me they found a dead tabby on the corner. It was so bad that the street cleaners wouldn't go near it. They had to call the city animal carcass cleaners to do it. I don't know if it was suicide or what. I thought cats knew three-dimensional space but apparently, they don't. I wasn't home when it happened and was thankful for that. Thank GOD. I was definitely in a shocked panic denial mode when I came home and he was missing. I went downstairs to ask the doorman.

"Did anyone mention seeing a cat in the hallway?" Denial comment number one.

"They found a cat on the street corner." The tears began to fall.

"The street cleaners found it and said it was so bad they had to call..."

"Don't say another word." Denial comment number two.

"Why did you leave your window open?" If I had any idea how to respond to that comment I would, but I didn't. I just repeated myself.

"I don't want to know anything. Please don't say another word and don't tell anyone. I don't want to be 'there's that woman in the building whose cat fell out the window.' I was the new girl in the building and knew that something of this nature would spread faster than my plummeting cat. The Cannon Ball. How perfect is that. The Cannon Ball. It only took a day or so before I ran into someone in the hallway.

"I heard about your cat." I didn't know who she was or how she knew or what to say. I was obviously "that" girl in the building who killed her cat. I realized being "that" girl was better than being "That" girl. So at that moment I decided to stick to my earlier decision to not sleep with anyone in the building. I had made that decision after hooking up with someone in another loft building down the street because I knew I would run into him again, which I did, and so the building, the street and anyone in a three mile radius was out. Downtown living. Downtown living. It was that small.

January 4, 2010 – WARD S

I found out there is an adolescent ward down the hall from me. I walk by it every morning. It must be a whole new world behind those doors. Adolescence is rough enough. Adolescence in a psych ward is another thing.

January 12, 2010 – DINOSAURS VERSUS EGGS

I'm starting to wonder more and more why the patients are so less sick here and I've come to one conclusion: the doctors here are old seasoned veterans of mental health treatment, whereas, at Ocean, the doctors were younger or newer to the system. Then there is the issue of residents. As a teaching hospital they give their opinions on treatment which the doctor can correct or tweak, but still. Some of them thought they knew it all and picked meds and dosage out of their conceited hair. It drove me nuts.

Hospital to hospital, medications do not run the same. I can say with no hesitation that Ocean over-medicates, period. There are no slugs in a bed in any of the wards here. But they do tend to conserve more here depending on what ward you happen to land in. I slowly realized that one of the doctors, the Dinosaur, was flipping the bird to the system and not adhering to the county pressure to move patients out even if they weren't ready. It was refreshing. He wasn't having "The Code" type of electric wet blanket draped across his back tell him what to do. He was here to rehabilitate the patient so they could get back out into the world without a twisting neck looking back at a voice on their shoulder. Both attendings did their old school job of practicing psychiatry despite the pounding stressors of the county to move them out. Move 'em out like cattle back to a non-promised land.

January 13, 2010 – RICKY RICARDO

His name was Ricky Ricardo, or at least that's what he liked to call himself.

"I'm festively plump. I dated the fridge when my boyfriend broke up with me."

"Why?"

"He wouldn't have sex with me so…I cut my wrist." He showed his wrist to me. It had a tiny white line.

"I couldn't do it all the way cause I was too drunk. I passed out in the middle."

"So you drink a lot."

"I used to."

"What about drugs?"

"Meth. But that was a long time ago."

"Your chart says you are bipolar with manic episodes."

"I go from straight into kinda this hypomanic state. I just want to have a steady life." I checked his chart and he had over 30 hospitalizations. He was 23 years old and it all started around 18. He was brought in on a 5150 for trying to stop a DUI investigation in Whittier. His friends were pulled over and he stepped in, made a scene, and they hauled him off to jail.

"I pretended to commit suicide with my shirt. I wrapped it around my neck and they saw the red marks and brought me here. I'd rather be here than in jail." He let out a loud bellowing laugh and shot me a grin-beaming smile.

"How do you like it here?"

"It's OK, better than jail. We have group every day but it doesn't do anything. We make a cup or a frog. It doesn't do shit for recuperation, just psychobabble bullshit." Ricardo admitted he knew he was bipolar. He also said he knew his meds and their milligrams.

"I finally have the right meds. Risperdal and Depakote." He was the first patient who knew his meds and their milligrams and actually liked them. He was Ricky Ricardo and he wasn't the first to do something to try and avoid having to do time in jail. Being behind bars in a tiny hole is worse than being locked behind closed doors inside a ward. At least you had group time to make frogs and color inside the lines, if you could, out of a children's coloring book.

Later that day I opened another case with PDNOS. PDNOS also had an interesting history. I was having trouble placing him and the IMI had some questions.

"Why has he gone from a hospital to jail to fishing to a hospital?" I had the feeling she wanted to know why he went fishing.

"Let me check with the doctor and I'll get back to you." The following day I brought up the plot of his life that seemed to cause a problem with placement.

"What do you want me to tell them?"

"Well, initially he was diagnosed with schizophrenia and he actually has schizoaffective disorder."

"So I'll tell them we were able to stabilize him with meds that could treat his evolving diagnosis."

"Yes." The doctor did his best to give an honest diagnosis but sometimes the story changed to fit the needs of a discharge. There were four different diagnoses in his chart and at this point the diagnosis would rest on how they could get him placed in an IMI, not what it actually was. He was a PDNOS, to a mood disorder, to paranoid schizophrenia, to a schizoaffective disorder patient. The IMI's only accepted three specific diagnoses: Chronic Paranoid Schizophrenia, Bipolar Disorder and Major Depressive Disorder with Psychotic Features. I wonder how you would feel with a chart that put a diagnosis in stone when that diagnosis wasn't actually the true diagnosis. What if the IMI would only accept an obsessive compulsive disorder patient this week? Would he magically become an OCD patient?

January 15, 2010 – THE BELLY DANCER

THE BELLY DANCER

She sleeps alone inside her bed
A thin white sheet floating above her head
Tucked down so it's there
And sometimes she's just
Lying on the side
Mouth closed

Sleeping
Like the only one who has never slept with her mouth closed

No drool.

The Belly Dancer was a 19-year-old girl. She was schizoaffective with manic episodes. She was also a poet.
"I write poetry. I'm really good." She smiled across her bed.
"You know manic people write great poetry. Have you written anything since you've been in here?"
"No. I can't. My brain is like a ruler. I have no creative energy. It's the Zyprexa. Zyprexa, it even sounds like a demon." Belly Dancer planned on teaching belly dancing in Venice to children when she was discharged, discharged in three days, so she thought.
"Do you know what a conservatorship is?"
"No. I don't understand that word." Opens Cases, a registered nurse from my office, was there to open up a case for me. Please don't explain to this poor girl what a conservatorship is; that she wouldn't be leaving in three days but might be stuck in a nightmare year of her pending life.
"A conservatorship means you have a person that is assigned to you. Like a guardian. And they help make decisions to do what's best for you."
"So, like a guardian. OK." She nodded her lice less head which thankfully after being shaved to the nines she was free from tiny menacing lines.
"I don't need anyone, I just need to get out of here." I ended the conversation for fear that Opens Cases would continue to spill the beans that no one had even opened in the ward. No one was going to explain conservatorship and leave a ward full of crazy screaming bodies ready to dismantle into a true nut job mode.
"We can talk more later." I got up and escorted Belly Dancer out the door. She was so sweet, smart, light and free. Free in spirit, and locked in her mind.

Later that afternoon I stopped by to see her. She was reading Hamlet.
"I love Hamlet." Her face lit up and she handed me her book. It was a comic storybook of Hamlet.
"That's really cool."
"I can read now."

"You mean you can read because your brain has slowed down."
"Yes, that's the only good thing about being here. I can read."

I thought of my first meeting with Sampson. It was a long extensive evaluation of my life and I remembered him asking me about books. "Can you read?" I didn't understand his meaning.
"Yes. I can read, but not really." Then he wrote a note in his hidden notebook resting comfortably on his knee.
"So, it's like I read a sentence, hello, how are you, and I read the hello and my brain skips to the you." I tried to explain.
"OK."

"So you've seen some positive results. You can read right?" I smiled at Belly Dancer, hoping she'd feel that same solace I did when I took my medication and could read an entire paragraph without a blur of my mind skipping fast forward.
"But everything slows me down. I don't like to be slow and still. I haven't written anything since I have been here."
"You should try. Your writing process may be different. Try and be aware of it. Maybe it won't run straight from the brain onto the paper, but you'll actually think about the words and where they fit on the page and make a sentence, you know?"
"Yeah." She nodded her head and I left it at that. I wrote my first poem the day I took my first medication. I thought I would somehow prove that medication didn't mean you couldn't be a poet. I've written hundreds of poems since. But I'll never know what I could have or would have written if I never did.

January 16, 2010 – COLUMBIA

I opened up another case today. Columbia was a 27-year-old who came to the states when she was 8 years old. She came to the hospital with lice and had a terrible blotchy hair cut which she didn't seem to mind because she spent the majority of her life with..
"Hair down to here." And she pointed to her hip.
"I like short hair." She said she had been in four hospitals and her mother was out to get her. She had visited a few times and had brought her some things.
"She gave me that over there." She pointed to a stuffed teddy bear

that looked like something she had had since childhood.

"Is that old?"

"No. It's not even mine." She said her mother told the police she said she tried to kill herself and that was why she was in the hospital.

"I never said that." She continued to tell me her story which was colorful and sad. Most of her hospitalizations were due to drugs, I think.

"So I did coke for a week because there was this guy who I liked and I wanted to get skinny for."

"I know what you mean, I have friends who do that." And I smiled without relaying the whole truth.

The truth being I tried to get skinny for Dean and cocaine fell in the mix of little food and wild wine. I thought that's what he wanted so I ran. I ran every day. I ran to avoid the crowd of fat that remained outside my belly button. Maybe I should have been a belly dancer instead.

I DO LINES OF COKE

I do lines of coke
And wonder why I can't feel anything.
Before a stabilizer
Now the lithium takes care of that.
I want to feel it.
So I cut more.
I want to be skinny
Stupid to think coke is going to thin me out
Fat chance.
I can't run like this
I'm a zombie with a flat brain.
How do I find an end when having answers should be enough?
Enough
A meaningless word
So I cut more
Hoping the speed of wit will find a home
Again
In my stale brain.

CHAPTER 26

JOURNAL ENTRY – ONE WORD: SHIT - 2006

Dean. His name was Dean and he was one word: Shit. I should have known the moment I drank his simmering smile cursed in red lips that he was timing my heart to fall. And it did. Sometimes there is a kinda hot that you feel in your ah..shit, beneath those Jesus Christ breaths and you're warming up in the toaster oven because you can hang with this kind of pride. This I know; he's hot and he knows he's hot and I am sufficiently hot to match his hot. If that is even hot enough. I knew I could get hot guys, but not this kind of hot. The kind of hot that makes you uncomfortable when it stands next to you in the elevator because heat from his body floats through the air and swirls around your skin and you're stuck in there for at least another floor hoping you can breathe enough to breathe. Sex. It started out being all about sex. It wasn't only about sex on my end, but I made it about sex in the middle of my mind cause it was a summer fling. It had to be a summer fling because he was leaving in the fall back to school. Carter introduced us one night at a party. They knew each other through home and grad school.

"The cab's here." We were all back at my place in West Hollywood and Dean tossed me an eyelash that asked if he was going to stay. Carter got up and walked toward the door.
"I'm going to stay." Dean stayed seated. I sat silent, not sure how Carter would handle the situation. Not sure how he was handling the situation. But he did. And that was the beginning of my summer sex fest all over the sweaty sheets with Dean. With Dean and his joints.

I thought my sleeping at his place every night which temporarily ended the Whole Foods trips and balcony sounds would piss Carter off. Or at least make him jealous. But it didn't. I saw no angry lip trying to tuck under a sad frown and it made me think, for the first time, maybe he wasn't in love with me deep down inside but didn't know what was inside. Or maybe I was wrong all these years. Yet, stuck in my head like fresh gum, I still somehow believed, truly believed, that he was still in love with me. He just didn't get it yet.

At some point I prayed I would get it.

WHAT'S A LOVE POEM WHEN YOU LOVE ALONE?

What's a love poem when you love alone?
It's glistening in your dreamy sun
An accomplishment
That he doesn't
Ask about.
It's a sad weird thing
Deep inside
You think
He thinks
Of you
Sometimes.

And you think of him all the time.

What's a love poem when you love alone?

It's thinking in between thoughts
About someone
A penetrating image
In your head
When you love alone
You continue to be there
With your thoughts
As you think it is
Or actually should be

It doesn't make it ours.

What's a love poem when you love alone?

It's a deep seated passion for someone beneath the unknown surface
That reeks taste.

Sex with Dean all summer was great. So was getting to know him
fast because we both knew we had a clock on our back. I fell for
him. I fell for him like a new fallen tree that hits a different bed of
rocks. Yes, I was still "that girl." I was the one waiting for the call.

I was the one coming over to his place. I was the one pulling the truth out of his gums. And then he was gone. Dean left and I was back with Carter like old times. Old times like old tears that never fled my eyes because at this point I didn't know what was going on. Dean would come and visit for interviews or to visit friends and we would sleep together. Hardcore sleep, and I would pretend that my heart was not burning my circulation. He would come and go and each time he left I would find a way to mentally make it more. My passion would continue to burn me at the stake. So I sat in the shower and let the water fall down and spark off my ear. But it didn't quit the ongoing thought of him, and our nights and why I still cared. But it felt good to feel in the shower. To breathe beneath the stream that warmed my face and fell across my lips and not in my mouth. I couldn't let the water into my mouth and clean out his soul. I couldn't stop the memories of our time together from this past weekend or the one I'd have two steps down the calendar map of who knows when. The shower was nice. The water felt good because it was synonymous with my feelings. Feelings that ran hard full and would fall onto the floor again and again into a drain. Every time I re-met him. Then he'd leave with a simple 'I'll call you' that never seemed to happen. But it didn't make me mad. Just disappointed. I gave him the benefit of so many doubts. I made assumptions on his behalf. I assumed he would get it. And it was my fault.

It was not enough, I was too plenty. The on and off was killing me. And the belief that he cared was worse than dropping a fresh mango down a dirty drain. I'd still stick my hand down there and pull out its smile. And the quiet sun would beam down on me but I couldn't feel it because I was already burned. The come and go, come and go, back and forth was driving my heart around a carousel. I would see him and I would want to cry. His walls would be up so I would have to hide the urge to press my body against his frame or else I would lose the game of love. No one would speak any truths and emotions would bubble up to the surface and it would burn. I begged myself not to cry because it would only make it real. I would focus on deep breaths to calm the storm that raged beneath my skin. But it was all such a lie. I knew I would fall apart. Alone. It was never goodbye because I was left with deeper ties made stronger by that silent sun. Distance made me think I was doing better until the memory would bark in my brain, taunting my heart.

The ins and outs of our sex never seemed to die. And my imagination would breed stupidity. One day he would love me. It would just take undying love, a perfect body, some more time, and I didn't know what the deal was. I'm a friend, he's my lover. No distinctions were ever made and the fear of hearing 'let's just be friends' would wreck all the work that I did. I thought, one more day and things will change. And all along I didn't know the waste of me.

When Dean would go back to school on the east coast things would resume with Carter. Resume spending almost every night together splashed with random times of sex with no warning or reached purpose. I guess we were friends with privileges. And I would wonder, does he remember my tits? Or the shape of my ass? He would come from behind and kiss the side of my neck and I would pray inside that my flimsy bones wouldn't melt beneath his mouth. I knew I'd been down this road to hell before, yet I was there. Today we were friends, then we were loosening the ropes that tied us into friendship. Walking backwards toward the bed I knew it would be easier than before. And I had certainty in uncertain hope that somehow things would be new. I'd forget the memory of promises to myself to stay away, and sex became a shadow hovering over wishful new love. And my old love would reignite and I would pray it was not fake for him. Just once. It's like he was groomed to be sickly alone. Like an encapsulated heart bleeding for love, not had, and still pounding.

So I guess you can say I was in some twisted non-love triangle. Neither of them wanted me officially, which left me with nothing. And I just wanted something. Out loud. I was myself, and it was scary for the men that crossed my path.

UNREQUITED LOVE II

How does it feel to burn in the sun?
To be the only one
To set fire to the heart
When your love is far apart.

FOR SOMETHING

Sometimes you have love
Sometimes you lose love
Sometimes you want love
And sometimes you don't want anything at all.

So when does it become something?

Does it fall from your tears
Into the drain
To become a stop
Of some sort of caring
Or does it simmer
In your restless sleep
Like a pot on the stove
Marinating in sauce
Bubbling at the surface?

You can keep it inside yourself
Like a jar
But love boils in the veins
And simmers to a pop
On the stove
So you have to put the lid on
To stop the hot splash
From searing your already warm self.

When it's fresh
It's something
When it's old
It's nowhere
When it's unclear
It's like driving through a forever car wash

As the water hits you hard
And the soap dusts the frame
And you wait for the cleansing
To the finish
To dry your tears
Of waiting
But you still may wait
For that love
For a love
For something.

CHAPTER 27

January 17, 2010 – WHAT'S THE NAME OF THE PLACE..WHAT'S THE NAME OF THE PLACE..WHAT'S THE NAME OF THE PLACE...

"My doctor said he was going to talk to me. He had a hearing yesterday and said conservatorship. I don't even know what that means."
"I think he is in a meeting right now but he will probably talk to you later." I didn't want to go there, nor should I go there.
"He said conservatorship can get me a place to stay when I leave."
"Yeah." I wanted out of the conversation so got outta there. A place to stay. It sound like it was some type of nice place and not some place that was locked and sick. Most of the patients didn't know the truth behind the walls they would soon reside in. And I was going to work with them on their discharge. Was I going to have to spend the next few weeks dancing around the truth while in the back of my mind I knew it was dark? The oxymoron of dark truth.

Sometimes the patients talked to each other and the ones that learned the term conservatorship had a paranoia mixed with a pleading disturbance that escalated them to *maybe* we should conserve to conservatorship status.
"I need to talk to you about your discharge plan." She was an older dark woman in her forties with three sharp teeth on the right side of her half hollow mouth and colorful beads from a necklace she made in recreational therapy.
"What's the name of the place..what's the name of the place..what's the name of the place...what's the name of the place...?" She shuffled down the hall with her shoelaceless sneakers in a frenzied panic and a sheet of glistening wet tears on the sides of her eyes that looked like saran wrap. She was searching her memory for the name of a shelter that a patient told her about when she strung her beads that chunked around her neck.
"A shelter?"
"Wait, wait here. Hold on." She shuffled fast but slow enough to keep her open shoes on and disappeared into the common room. I

waited and she popped back onto the catwalk.

"New Day. It's called New Day." New Day was a common shelter we used when we discharged patients and it was becoming a new buzzword on the ward for freedom.

"You need to calm down." I heard earlier in rounds that the Dino was thinking of conservatorship. She was one of many walking down the plank to a bottomless ocean. She stopped and faced me.

"Please don't let them put me on conservatorship." The patients were talking, and the deteriorating mental health from the idea of a forever locked placement was only making them walk down the plank farther to the end of life on earth. She shuffled away in her long gray braids and continued. "What's the name of the place...what's the name of the place...what's the name of the place."

January 19, 2010 – BOLD FACE LIES

It was a bold face flat out lie.

"I don't know when you are going."

"Well I have a friend and I can't find her number and I know I can stay with her, I just need her number. Can you get that for me? My 14 day hold is up tomorrow so I have to get out of here." I was surprised she knew her hold was up but didn't know that she was facing a court hearing that would lead to a conservatorship.

"I'm not sure what the plan is, but the doctor should have some answers for you after tomorrow."

"Will you tell him I would like to speak to him? I wrote him a letter and he hasn't come to talk to me."

"I'll tell him you asked about him." Another lie. Later that day I called her HIH for younger adults, and they had lost touch with her about a month ago. They were relieved that she was OK. Being in the hospital was OK, I suppose.

"I don't want to talk to them. I don't need therapy, I am getting that here. I will see them maybe when I get out." Her therapist wanted to come out that day but I told her to wait. I didn't want to lose the trust I had managed to build the past week and tomorrow was a whole new day. She was going to have a whole new future ahead of her and having a therapist she didn't think she needed caught up in the mix would only make me lose my thin ice footing.

January 10, 2010 - ORANGES

I bought a new juicer recently. I've wanted one for quite some time and was so excited I kinda went overboard. I made my way to the produce district east of the skyscrapers listed downtown and bought a HUGE box of oranges that have been sitting on my stove for almost two weeks. Every time I walked into my loft a rush of oranges sitting in cardboard hit my face so I decided to bring some to the hospital. I made my way through the security doors and offered some oranges to the guards. Then I hit up the nursing station where they were gratefully dispersed. An old woman standing outside the glass watched as the oranges were distributed one by one. I was ready to hit up the next station in the other ward when I was stopped. She stood in front of me when her tiny old blotchy skinned hands held out to me and her pleading eyes cried without tears.

"Can I give one to the patient?" I never knew what they could or could not have because some had diet restrictions, plus it didn't seem fair to give one thing to one patient and not have enough to offer to the rest of them.

"She can have it." I handed her the orange and she bowed in gratitude. Later that day I dropped off my usual Vanity Fair magazine in the common room in one of the other wards. It was their turn to get it and the next time I donated some clothes they would be left in that ward as well. I tried to rotate the wards with gifts so I did in some respect think I was being fair.

CHAPTER 28

January 23, 2010 – TEN YEARS LATER

Ryan knocked on my door today. I opened the door and there he was. Standing there, ten years later.

"Jesus Christ, Ryan?" He picked me up and hugged me.

"I'm heavy." But I looked good. Quite good, thank God. I had just gotten home from work on a Friday and had a nice blue dress on and my hair was straightened, thank God.

"Erica."

"What are you doing here?"

"I'm visiting a friend here and wondered if you were living in LA, so I looked you up and called your parents' house and spoke to your mom."

"Come in." I walked into my living space and he checked out the place.

"Your place is nice."

"Thanks. Can I get you anything?" I walked over to the fridge like it was easy as pulling out a chair before you sat down. It was weird. I was old. Or life had been through me so much that I was free of obsessional thoughts of another time. Another person. I was another person. And I was waiting for something to reach my cool steady heeled walk. It was weird.

"I'm good." I opened the fridge and took out a Stella.

"I'll have one if you are."

"Yeah, I think I need a beer for this." He sat down in one of my chairs and I sat across the room.

"You look great." He looked at me up and down and I knew he meant it.

"So you called my mom."

"Yeah, last night. She gave me your number." I thought about last night, how I was watching TV and my phone rang and it was my mom but I didn't feel like talking so didn't pick it up. Then it rang again with a number I didn't recognize so didn't pick it up either. I knew I had messages on my voicemail but hadn't checked them yet.

"I called you last night and left a message."

"I haven't checked my voicemail. Jesus Ryan, it has been like ten years." He nodded.

"I didn't know if you were married with children or what, but I knew I had to see you." It was straight out of a movie. He continued.

"I'm sorry I've been such a bad friend. I've thought about you on and off the past ten years but never tried to reach you. I'm sorry about that." I felt nothing.

"It's fine. I didn't expect you to keep in touch after graduation and that night."

"That night was very special. We had some great sex. I think there was a lot of pent up energy that needed to be released." I wasn't embarrassed because I was too surprised that I wasn't surprised that he was sitting in my loft and saying these things.

"I want you to know that I've always had feelings for you and have thought about you over the years." Why God, whyyy.

"I'm sorry I lost touch."

"No need to apologize. I expected you to lose touch because throughout college I always was the one that came to you. We probably wouldn't have been friends if it weren't for me." It was a truth and it swallowed out of my tongue with no hesitation.

"I'm sorry about that. I always cared about you even if I didn't show it."

"Okay." I half believed him. The rest of me was uncertain.

"So are you single?"

"Yeah, I'm living the bachelor life and love it."

"Get this, I was engaged." He nodded his head up and down like even he was surprised. I wasn't.

"Oh, how did that go?"

"I broke it off. She wasn't...she was lame. I broke it off six months ago. And haven't been with anyone since."

"How long are you here for?" I was so amazed by my nonchalant coolness it was hard to believe myself.

"I leave in three hours."

"How long have you been here in LA?"

"A week. I've been visiting my friend Jay." A week. A week and he shows up at my door three hours before take off.

"I would have contacted you sooner. I don't know why I didn't. I'm sorry. I hope you can forgive me." I didn't know why he didn't contact me the last ten years and why I didn't care. I was that used to men disappointing me that I didn't get disappointed anymore.

"There's nothing to forgive. It's fine."

"I want to have you in my life. I want you to come visit me."

"Maybe. Let's get out of here. I'm going to use the bathroom then we'll go." I got up and he glanced over to the table. One of my poetry books was sitting on the table. He picked it up and breezed through it.

"Wow. This is a lot of poetry."

"Yeah." I got up and walked toward the kitchen to put my sucked down Stella on the counter.

"Here. There's one in here about you." I took the book and flipped till I found the page.

"Here. Read it. I'm going to use the bathroom then we'll go." I bounced it on the table in front of him. He looked at the book with his hesitant eyes and I walked toward the bathroom. I knew he was nervous to read the work and was more shocked then ever that I wasn't. This is me here. Take it as it should have been all those years. Not a scared fist not ready to let the fingers go into a hand. But a woman living her life with poetry to stand by it. I returned from the bathroom and sat back in my chair. His face was still forward in the book and he sipped another bottle of Stella.

"Wow." He looked up and read everything I felt about everything that didn't happen in college and his reaction was in 3-D all over his lashes.

"You ready to go?" I walked up, took the book, and put it back in its place.

"I'm sorry I never told you how I felt in college."

"It's cool. Really. Let's go." And it was, for some reason. I'm sure the intensity of my words on the page of a poem titled "Ryan" was sending some kind of numb blender through his chest but I didn't know so didn't care. I didn't know what I felt or why I didn't seem to feel much. I had turned into the guy sitting across from me now. The guy that never told me anything. Never said a word about being a great friend or wannbe lover or whatever. What did I expect? I didn't expect no words, no thoughts, nothing to call my own. As I sat there.

We finished our beers and left. We walked to Olvera Street and had lunch. The plots of our lives had changed so much over the years yet our connection remained. Three hours later it was time to say good-bye. It was time for that awkward moment. We never really kissed before. Our sex was lipless for the most part, and now it was a whole new game.

"OK, well bye." I gave him a quick hug with no lingering moment so the awkward are we going to kiss second wouldn't expand into a bumping mouth road.

"You have to come visit."

"Maybe I will."

Three weeks later, I did.

February 15, 2010 – YOU DO BETTER ON THEM

My mom told me to stay on my meds because "you do better on them." In other words, you can't be fine without them. It's the same thing, an adamant soft strong knowing voice that softly speaks right. She's right. But I think otherwise. I think maybe I can do without as much as 200 milligrams and do with 150, like it makes that much of a difference.
"You have to take your medicine. You have to take it. You do better on it." She's my mother so I guess she knows what I do better on than not. And I've been fighting the truth. Her truth, which is the truth if I've ever known one.

It's always the same conversation when I go there.
"You have to stay on your meds." I never ask why she thinks that but I kinda knew.
"OK, OK."
She hears the pulse of I don't think I want to speak in between the pauses and the mantra continues.
"You have to stay on your meds." With a bipolar mother that was never medicated, she knew what life was like inside the vein of insane.

It's so strong and about-face that there is no room to think otherwise, nor should there be, because her tone and statement of truth reeks belief.
"I might just do better without them" never crossed my lips but it breathed beneath my truth. But I know I don't have the guts to do otherwise. And the voice of her telling me so hard, so seriously, without a pop in the air of a sentence…
"You have to stay on your meds."

It kills me. When I go there and that's the known know.

TRUTH

I love that I have someone
Other than myself
To tell me the truth
And know the truth
Every time
Every truth is every time.

In all the dying truth
In the world
She is the vein that
Keeps it alive
It takes a lot of guts
To survive
In this world
While breathing honesty

And she made it mine.

CHAPTER 29

February 19, 2010 – PICK ONE…

I had to go to the psychiatrist today for my check in.
"How long have I been on Lamictal...one and a half, two years?" Sampson flipped through his diary, actually my diary, and looked up.
"Three years." My stomach hurt, I think. I don't really recall because that's what happens when a person goes into shock.
"Three years!! Do I have to worry about long term side effects?"
"No." I didn't believe him. I thought of that quote from Belly Dancer, "I'm not going to take some medication for ten years and wake up one day with a tic in my back. It's not normal to take the same medication all that time...every day." Actually it's twice a day and now I was counting.
"What are some problems people have discovered?"
"Some people don't like how it slows them down, some get constipation." Wait, constipation? Forget about being slowed down, I was used to that and had no idea what that other life of speed was like.
"So maybe it's not the blue, feta and Parmesan cheese that is my diet, it could be the meds." I didn't expect a reply.
"OK. Never mind."

After my appointment, I picked up Smooth Move herbal tea. Out of all the potential problems that could arise from the Lamictal I was worried about not being able to shit because maybe that would mean it would be harder for me to ever lose weight like the rest of the world. But just like the slowing down effect, at this point I wouldn't know if I was constipated. Who's to say I had just become accustomed to it by now..??!

Later that night I gave some thought to the long list of meds that I had taken over the years. Some stood out in my mind when I thought of serious detrimental side effects that entailed terrible work on my part to recover from. First was the lithium. Lithium was mercury on the brain and lard on my back. I managed to gain 30 pounds in about a month, and it's not something that simply comes off when you stop taking it. I had to run and run and run on the cement sidewalks of Los Angeles. You can imagine what it must have been like to run with 30 extra pounds. I couldn't imagine it till I was actually there pounding the pavement, literally. It was like carrying dumbbells on my shoulders and the weight ran down to my knees. Weight that ruined my mind and plummeted me into depression, making me want to die.

"I'd rather be crazy and skinny than fat and sane" jumped out of my mouth when I made an appointment to see Sampson, because enough was enough fat on my ass. He got it. It was too bad that I got it too late. I came from a family obsessed with weight and fitness. Forget about *me* trying to recover from that lard pumping place in my life, I don't think *they* ever recovered from that period of time in my life either because ever since then they would make positive comments about my weight. All the time.
"You look good." Blah blah blah. Eventually the lithium also took hold of my hands and they would shake pretty hard. I would go out to sushi with my dad and couldn't use chop sticks to pick up my food cause my hands would shake so hard the fish would just fall right through the sticks. Must have been pretty uncomfortable for them. Forget about me. Comfort at that point was a childhood dream like thinking heaven was sleeping on a marshmallow bed with laps of chocolate sheets. All and all, lithium was a shitty beast that managed to ruin my life for about a year. Then there was Trileptal.

Trileptal was an antipsychotic and seizure medication which was interesting, cause I wasn't psycho and never had a seizure in my life, but I figured that I had a hypomanic brain that was pretty much constantly having some mild seizure so it made sense that it worked to calm my mind. But like any drug, overtime, it developed side effects. Trileptal made me shake. It would randomly send electric shocks throughout my body when I slept which didn't hurt but was disturbing because I would have a jumping jolt out of nowhere. It was like involuntarily sticking my finger in an electric socket periodically throughout the night, jolting myself awake so I ended up sleeping here and there until the next jolt shook my insides and jumped my outsides inside my calm sheets. One time I slept over at a guy's house who I was thinking about dating and in the morning he said that I must have had some wild dreams or nightmares because I would shake every now and then throughout the night. That pretty much was the final straw to pull the plug of the electric socket that I lived in.

Then there was Effexor. Effexor was an anti-depressant and mood stabilizer that I stopped suddenly because I thought it contributed to my weight gain and I didn't know when you stop Effexor all at once, you would experience this weird sound in your head like a muffled noise that hits your brain every few times an hour. It scared some of the shit out of me but I was determined to stop any meds that were potentially going to contribute to my pregnant looking flabby stomach or ballooned double watermelon ass. Then there was Wellbutrin.

Wellbutrin was an anti-depressant. It would keep me alive and alert in the morning but at night I would float sleep. Float sleeping was like lying alone on a boogie board in the middle of the ocean not fully asleep, and not totally awake. It was like slightly getting wet here and there as the waves rocked your body back and forth, and I would sort of remain dry and sort of wet at the same time until the sun came up and would beam down on my tired limbs and mind causing me to have to face the blazing day. It was terrible. So I decided to try Wellbutrin SR. Wellbutrin SR had a slow release after you took it in the morning. I would be in rounds and feel it trickle into my blood stream causing a slow blurry moment that would pass over a long tick tock clock period. I would have to fight to appear normal and pray none of the doctors noticed the wave of drag that ran through my veins.

Then there were some others randomly tossed in there in the trying dump tank. Seroquel, for example. Tried it, hated it. I tried to stay away from the drugs that were smiling on the television with a quick speed voice of side effects. That part didn't really bother me as much as the woman walking in the forest with a blue tint to represent the dismal color of depression. I was waiting for the commercial that had fluorescent colors shooting out of the antennae as a manic person ran through the woods, laughing merrily, with no self control. There was no commercial for my condition. My condition wasn't on the map because it held such a small percentage of the population. I just wanted to be normal. And sometimes it worked for a day. Then the voice made its presence, again.

Ostracizing me from the pack of the world. I would fall to my knees crying that no pill would make a difference. But I take it and say to myself I am the same, like everyone else in their mind. But it never goes so far. I am only me.

CHAPTER 30

February 28, 2010 – CANDY CART

An obese patient whaled up to me today begging me for chips, sugar, something to curb her preservative withdrawal.

"I don't think they can give out candy and stuff." His blob face sat sad. It then occurred to me that at Eastside Memorial there was no candy cart. Ocean had a lady to stroll down the ward like a 7/11 on wheels, and here there were no cheetos or milk duds. Nothing. It seemed to suck for the patients but I had a flash of those patients' faces that would stare at the cart rolling by and could only watch it roll by because their pockets ran dry. Some had to decide if they were going to spend their quarters on cigarettes or on snickers or on the pay phone to someone who may or may not pick up. I wondered if patients would trade sex for money. Especially those that were really hard up on cigarettes. Sex on the ward seemed to be impossible, but it happened. Sometimes there was rape late at night. A remember a patient at Ocean once told me another patient crawled into his roommate's bed and raped him. And reporting it was met with an eye roll like it was a lie. Just like Skid Marks soup dispenser story that got her kicked out of her board and care. According to the rest of the non crazy world, the truth rarely, if ever, sat in the teeth of a patient. The patient's story was just that. A story.

March 4, 2010 – MEDICAL CASE WORKER II

It was time for my promotion. After a year as an MCW I could graduate to an MCW II. Same job. More pennies. I filled out all the paperwork and, once again, was faced with that box you check about your criminal history. Misdemeanor. Felony. It's the same old stop, pause, and question yourself...do I check the box yes? I didn't. I figured if I made it through the first round of background checks (the other one being the drug test that I managed to pass thanks to the Q Carbo 32 grape drink I guzzled to mask the thc in my urine) then there wouldn't be another test. I was wrong. I received a phone call a few weeks later from human resources stating that I had lied on my application. I went on to explain that it was an oversight. Lie. And said I would disclose all the info about my misdemeanors. Both a DUI and driving with a suspended license. Turns out, I didn't lie on the initial application and had thankfully written a saga about the whole mess but since I forgot about my disclosure I managed to come up with another lie on the spot.

"Yeah, since I disclosed that info the first round I didn't think I had to do it again."

"You always have to disclose information regardless of your employment status."

"Oh OK. Thanks for telling me. I'll make sure I'll check that box from now on." He bought it, but I still had a warning and was filed with a drunk driving flag on my back. I was pissed but knew I deserved it. It had been five years now, and counting, and my DUI continued to pop up. Five down and five more to go!

March 5, 2010 – QUANTITY NOT QUALITY

Jesus hell Mary Maria. My office is coming down on me to open more cases.

"So it's about quantity not quality."

"No Erica, it's about quality care. The more patients you work with the more quality care they can get."

"So if I open two cases and spend two hours with each of them that's 4 hours. If I open 1 case and spend 4 hours with them than it's the same billing, right?" There was no logic to any answers.

"You need to open 10 cases."   I had a new supervisor who I was going to kill. I missed a meeting and she said she was going to write me up. FUCK THAT. I already had two strikes on my record for lying about the DUI and driving with a suspended license and now she wanted to write me up for missing a meeting? I knew I was going to lose the quality versus quantity care conversation so let it go. Fuck her.

March 6, 2010 – NO JUSTICE FOR ANYONE

So I opened a new case today. Not Knowing.

"Do you know what conservatorship is?"

"I get to go to a place. I went to court and I told the judge I wanted to be conserved because they told me if I did that then I could leave the hospital and go to a place." Well that may be the worse lie yet announced in what is supposed to be a just environment. Justice for all!! Unless you were mentally ill. They were easy to manipulate and toss into a system of grim and sour cheese.

"Yes, you will have a place to go. It will be a locked facility." News to him.

"It's a mental place?"

"Yes."

"Do I get to go to the movies and beach and stuff?" I don't even have words to describe my thoughts and once again was not going to go there. I took out my notebook and drew a picture to explain the process of referrals and said that I didn't have all the details about the places but that those facilities would come interview him and tell him everything he needed to know and answer all his questions. I wanted to die but thought that was the best thing to do. I still don't know what's worse. Knowing the whole truth of the future of your terrible locked life with movies you could watch in the mental infested common room and having to deal with that thought every day until it was time to go? Or not know and get there and find out. No news is good news, right?

Later I went to do an HIH referral for Axis II.

"I was beat up at the other hospitals so I am scared."

"I'm sorry. I know that probably happens sometimes."

"No one believed me." And they never ever did and never will.

"Do you still hear the voices?"

"Yes."

"How often?"

"All the time."

"Do you hear them now?"

"Yes, just not as loud."

"What do they say?"

"You're fucking stupid. You're an asshole."

"I always hear patients say the same thing, they hear harsh things, curse words."

"Yeah. People tell me in here they hear the same thing. This one girl walks around and calls herself a bitch. I told her not to say that because it's not true and it's the voices."

"That's nice of you. So the people aren't that bad here?"

"They're better than the other hospitals I've been in." He had been in 5 different hospitals in the last year. 5 hospitals with 20 different medications and still…the voices kept coming.

March 9, 2010 – HE'S HONEST…OF COURSE HE'S HONEST

I checked in with Axis II today. I am thinking about opening a case on him because I think he is going to be here awhile, plus I like him. He's honest.

"There are ways to kill yourself in here."

"Like how?" He sat with his legs squatting on a chair and pointed to the ceiling.

"I can break that light."

"But it's plastic."

"But the bulb's not." I didn't think he was going to do a Spiderman spring out of his chair and do anything and was happy he was honest with me. Honest about his suicide attempts, his voices, his fears and his life.

On my way out I ran into Smiles. He asked if I could give his girlfriend a letter for him.

"Who's your girlfriend?"

"She's on the other ward. We met at smoke break and talk every time." I wondered if she thought he was her boyfriend and thought about asking her next time I was on that ward. Maybe.

March 12, 2010 – HER PLAN

Belly Dancer left today. Her hold was up and she walked out the door. Her mom tried to get her to go home with her but she wasn't having it. We gave her bus tokens and she is noted as being discharged to self. I thought of a meeting I had with Belly Dancer and the Dinosaur. He had asked her to write a letter that mapped out a clear, coherent, pragmatic plan for her life. Her plan to teach belly dancing in Venice and live by the beach in a bush if her friend didn't take her in wasn't good enough for him. He spent an hour trying to convince her that her plan was not linear, that her thoughts didn't make sense and that they were all over the place. She cried and cried and kept repeating herself.

"You aren't listening to me. I have a plan. I'm going to live with my friend Evan on Santa Monica Blvd. I might start school at Santa Monica College in the fall and I'm going to teach kids dancing." It sounded like a plan to me, but not to the Dino. He asked her to go back to her room and think about what he said and write down a plan and not something that was "all over the place." When the Dino got the note he said it was interesting. Not clear, not linear, and not anything near what he wanted to hear after his attempt to make her be someone else, have a future of someone else and live a life of something else. But her hold was up and she was ready to go. She'll be on the streets in Venice by sunset and start teaching her belly dance classes on the boardwalk come Sunday.

YOUR UNORGANIZED THINKING WILL BE REJECTED

When you're too this
Or that
Or not enough
For him
Or her
But still standing
Every day
On your feet
And thinking
Inside
Your own head
And springing
True thought
From disorganized thinking

You will be rejected.

The Dino also asked another patient, Wheelchair, to write a list of 15 things he would do not to come back to the hospital.
"Can you speak to me for a minute?" I was on my way to see another patient when he stopped me.
"Can you help me with this list." He wheeled his crocked legs over to a table that had a dictionary he used to make lines on a page.
"Not use drugs." Was number one, the only number on the list. His sad 21-year-old years stared up at me. I was afraid to tell him what to write and for him to not be able to take credit for it so slowly pulled answers out of his chair.
"Where do you see yourself in 5 years?"
"Making money."
"What is your dream?"
"I wanna work at Wal-Mart."
"Good. Write that down." He continued with his list and was able to come up with the remaining 13 pleas to get out. Get out of the wheelchair, get counseling, spend time with his nieces and nephews. The list was good. He didn't spell any words close to him getting out of that chair any time soon but at least he had a plan to show the Dino. Jumping off an impasse left him in the chair. Getting out of it would be a problem. He wasn't from LA County so technically we couldn't conserve him, but I had seen other patients manage to

slip through the county system and end up in a non-residential ward cell. I prayed he could return to his family in his known county and they would take him back. As of now, they had no intention of allowing his wheelchair back in their house and preferred to leave it out on the curb. Which they did. Where it would get stolen. The clock was ticking. Without a discharge plan in place in a week or so the papers would be filled and he would end up here in LA, in his wheelchair alone and wondering if writing down his Wal-Mart dream would ever come to fruition.

Earlier that day I touched base with Axis II. I had made an HIH referral for him and they were there the next day.
"I'm not sure I want to do this. Let me think about it." I thought it was a legitimate request and then realized that this guy had been hospital surfing the past year. He would be discharged, then walk to another hospital and turn himself into the psych ER.
"I'm going to kill myself." When I asked him his plan if he didn't decide to do HIH he said the same thing.
"I'll kill myself." He said he needed time for the medication to work and then would think about HIH when his head was clear.
"When do you think that will be?"
"I don't know."
"Well you can't stay here forever."
"If I agree to the plan does that mean I will be discharged sooner?" He didn't realize that statement stamped him with a player notice on his head. I knew he was a waste of HIH's time and was mad that I actually thought he wanted help. He didn't want outside help. He wanted inside care. Food, shelter, group, TV, immediate friends that beat to the same drum. To him, this was the Eastside Hotel.

March 16, 2010 – THE LIGHT BULB

My new supervisor, ah…no. She is this short round woman that was shaped like a light bulb with bright red roots that spilled out onto her fake dyed hair. She had a power trip and I wasn't having it.
"I have your evaluation papers for you to sign." She pulled out the papers to officially make me a MCW II. I really didn't give a shit

about the title but sure wasn't going to have her pull a power trip on me.

"Should I read it to you or do you want to read it?"

"I can read…it." Bitch. I started to skim the paragraphs assessing my performance and began to slow down.

"Fails to complete all required meetings." And there was a box that had a check mark that said I also failed to take instruction or listen to my supervisor. It was something like that. What the fuck balls.

"Ah, you wrote me up for missing that meeting?"

"Well I did tell you I was going to put it in your evaluation."

"Yeah and I did say I was going to fight it. I'm not signing this."

"You still passed probation."

"I don't care. This is ridiculous." We started going at it and I was surprised at my hardcore stance and ability to stand up for myself.

"I can't believe after almost two years of hard work I am getting written up for missing a meeting." I didn't even care to address the Ocean section that stated that one of the reasons I left Ocean was due to "conflicts with interpersonal relationships." 'Relationshipssss' – plural. I had one person, The Demon, who I had conflict with. Not two. But I was so focused on that goddamn missing meeting clause and checked box saying I didn't take commands that I left the Ocean bullshit out.

"I was actually being nice by only adding the missed meeting. You have also been late turning in your time card."

"WHAT?" I hoped my face actually said what the FUCK!

"If you want I can add that to the paragraph."

"Why would I want you to add it to the evaluation?" I called her supervisor in and addressed the clause. Her supervisor had told me weeks before that if the meeting thing came up on the evaluation she would take care of it then. Her signature was on the evaluation so she obviously wasn't going to take care of anything. I was thrown under the bus not more or less but period.

"Let's just say what this is really about. You are trying to establish boundaries and have some power trip thing going on here and this is your way of making a point."

"No. This is about you not doing what you are asked to do. I did tell you I was going to write it up."

"I understand that, and I did tell you that I thought it was ridiculous and I still think this is ridiculous but am being bombarded by both of you here so I guess I'll just have to let it go." I fought my ass off to keep the tears from falling down my watery eyes. Thank God I kept them in my eyeballs and not outside running down my face onto my knee-high socks. I got up and left to finish the rest of the paperwork. When I came back to hand it to the light bulb she was still in the room with her supervisor. Laughing, smiling, probably cleaning up the mess we just had by putting herself in the spot light. She was a bulb. She didn't need a light on her ass. I was sure her previous corporate America trash shoot job taught her how to kiss ass and work the structured hierarchical bullshit of American business politics just fine. She looked over the paperwork and saw that I checked a box no for the question, 'have you ever had any criminal history?' She made a cautious face toward her supervisor who was fake fiddling around on the printer and it was clear. Her supervisor told her about my misdemeanors and probably said that is why I was being sensitive to any negativity on my evaluation. Have you ever been committed of a crime IN HEALTH CARE! Can YOU read motherfucker!

I walked out. Ten minutes later when the clock allowed my release from a prison of bullshit I ran into her in the hall.
"I like your socks, it is very hot on the runway right now." What?
"Oh, thanks."
"So are we good?"
"Yeah...I still disagree but I am glad we had it out." Her face shot a wave of crinkle through her skin like I just said something weird and offsetting. But the truth always does, especially when you adhere to the politically correct nuances of office life. Barf.
"OK, well bye." It would be a longggg road with this bitch and I would have to find a way to deal I think by not dealing. I was smarter than her and would find a way to drive her mad. Kill her with kindness? Maybe. We shall see. Bitch.

March 28, 2010 – LOVE INSIDE LOCKED DOORS OUTSIDE

I met Smiles girlfriend on the Ward today. She was fat and sweet. She had a paper airplane letter in her hand that she was planning on giving to Smiles.
"He's so sweet. My last girlfriend broke both my ribs."
"So you were a lesbian?"

"Well, both."

"Oh."

"So Smiles told me about you. He said you are really nice and can get me into Sunny Side."

"Well..not exactly. Is your sister your conservator?"

"Yes, she is the only one that helps me."

"I might want to speak with her."

"I can give you her number."

"I'll get it from you next week." I might open a case on her, but would have to get a signature from her sister since she was the conservator. I would also have to be careful not to become the middleman between the two lovers. Both Smiles and his girlfriend were gunning for Sunny Side. The treatment team wanted to keep them apart and I knew that down the road I would have a say in whether she would go to an IMI or Sunny Side. I recalled Preggers wanting to return to Sunny Side to be with her boyfriend. And now these two wanted to go there and be together.

If it were me, I would want to go somewhere I could be with someone I liked, or could potentially love.

March 29, 2010 – THE HOARDER

Yes, I opened another case today. The Hoarder. She was a flashback to Trader Joes. She was an old lady with silver hair and the same mantra.

"I don't need to be here. They took me here after I was stabbed three times." She pointed to her elbow, then pulled up her leg to show another scab, then stuck her finger up her nose.

"They stabbed me here too." She was a sweet lady who, like Trader Joes, had worked as a schoolteacher in the Los Angeles County Public School District. She pulled out a plastic bag with a stack of papers with things scribbled on different sheets of paper. Her penmanship reminded me of Trader Joes, as did her inability to accept why she was brought into the psych ER. I found out in rounds that she was a hoarder. She had not paid her gas bill in two years and had piles upon piles of crap all over her tiny apartment. Trader Joes and The Hoarder. Hoarders. Big time.

Erica Loberg

March 30, 2010 – A CEMENT BLOCK

"She says she has a migraine but there is no way to prove it. There's no test you can take to show any migraine exists." The doctor was trying to treat a patient that Excedrin, Tylenol, Ibuprofen or any other medication couldn't handle.

"Maybe she thinks too hard." It was my only explanation to a problem that had no answers in the medical field. I thought of my childhood of festering horrific migraines that didn't have any hard hat to protect me. It was like someone poured cement into my head and it turned into a hard block that would swing back and forth inside my brain, hitting the insides over and over and over. BAM BAM. The block would ricochet off all sides of my brain leaving no relief, no position to sleep in or comfortable pillow to rest on. My parents didn't understand that it was not a headache, not a migraine, it was an indescribable death with no end. My mom would sit by my bed and put a cold cloth on my forehead to soothe the pain which was like trying to have water penetrate a cement block. And there was no way to prove it, or show the amount of pain that occurred more than often throughout my childhood. I think I thought too much. And it ended in a mind beating inside a cage.

This patient had a headache, or migraine, either way, the mind needed some help outside a laboratory mixing chemicals to make a Tylenol pill. Maybe medical marijuana was the answer.

CHAPTER 31

JOURNAL ENTRY – DOUBLE DIPPED INTO A DUMP 2006

EXTERIORS ARE VOID

You're too thin.
That's why
You spent a year and a half turning thin
You're too thin.
Your soft ghostly rolls
Like a horse who knows his saddle.
Having sex
Fat awareness ruins the chance of attention to your sex life
Are my arms fat?
You're too thin.
You can bite me.
Your red shades don't fool anyone.

Exteriors are void.

Dean dumped me today, over the phone.
"You're too skinny." Thank you. Was the first thing that came to my head.
"Ah...what?" I didn't know what to say. After a year of busting my ass to be skinny for him only to find out THAT was the reason he never committed to me sent me over the edge. Over-The-Edge. Of course I starved myself weeks before he came into town and ran. And ran some more. Of course I sucked in every line of oxygen and pretended I was fine only to make my stomach flat. I was not skinny, I was normal.
"You're too skinny."
"Is that why you didn't sleep with me the last time you were in town?"
"Yeah. I'm sorry." The pounding of my heart starting to beat up my throat and shot lightening into my eyes that sprayed down my face. I had no words to describe the shock that I thought would mask the pain but the depth was too strong. It was time. I went for it.

"Anorexia runs in my family and you have the gull to tell me I'm too skinny when I am the normal healthy one?!" As if the nightmares of growing up surrounded by skinny slims and always thinking you were fat and now finally being thin was not biting my face off.

"That's the only thing." He said with a blank silence that followed. I held the silence not knowing what to be. I was ready to pull the string of fairness. I did what any logical person does, I hit back. Below the belt.

"Ok." And that was my big response that was only a punch to my insides because I didn't know how to go below the belt.

"I have to go." The click happened before I could hear it.

"Wait... What?" And he hung up before I could stop my shaking throat.

I hung up and hysterically balled. What?! You'd think I would be like "Thank you. Thanks for calling me skinny." But it all seemed so ridiculous. And to think the last time he was here he slept in my bed and didn't lay a fingernail on me while I lied there thinking I was skinnysexy. Fucccckkkk that.

Two minutes later I picked up the phone to his voicemail and left a message, something about OK, that's fine, I'm sorry... It's all a blur but I think I was trying to pretend that didn't just happen and the flipping coin that was my mind had landed on a heads up, you're too thin and I tried to flip it over and make a tale instead of a truth. But it was already on the floor. It was too late. It was definitely not okay. And I never heard from him again. At least I didn't think I would.

I DIDN'T KNOW

I never really knew about unrequited love
It sounded so unsettling
Yet everyone uses it to describe sad love that is one sided
Not returned
Burning a hole in the bridge of exchange
And I didn't even know

You give not to receive.

Carter also dropped out of my life. Faster and swifter than The Cannon Ball did.

After a year of best friendship Carter moved back to his homeland. He dropped off the planet just like he always did when we weren't in the same city. Six months later I heard that his father passed and called him to give my condolences. I was hurt and surprised that he didn't call me and tell me himself. He inherited an island of money and moved to another country to take over his father's business. And like forever mine, I would never know if that would be that.

I knew it wasn't my mental illness that kept men away because I didn't really talk to any of them about it. Maybe it was the way I was because of the disease. I was over the top. Not mainstream. Hardcore and honest to a truth that most people couldn't handle. I was the girl that didn't cry wolf cause you're a step before the fangs. You would think my psychiatrist would give up by now on the question that he has asked for five years now.

"Any love interest?"

"No. Still single." All aspects of my life seemed to be on board with normalcy except that one.

"I actually prefer to be alone. Cuts down on the drama." I knew that was the truth but didn't know if I preferred to be alone because I had become accustomed to it so I didn't know anything else or what. I'm sure deep hypnosis would reveal that I was damaged from the clothesline of disappointments and rejections. At the end of the line I would always be rejected. When Ryan showed up and apologized for not being with me in college and for losing touch over the decade I didn't feel much. I was softly numb and happy it didn't deeply affect me. It meant I was over that phase of my life, or I was so wounded that I managed to find a way to turn myself off. I can't be 100% sure of what I'll feel if Carter reappears in my life. And I wasn't 10% sure if he ever would. I do know that I did worry if any day would come that I would have a serious relationship. When would I tell him that I was manic depressive? What would he say, think, do? Would he want to have children with a person that could pass on a mental disease? These were questions that I wasn't ready to ask but didn't have to. Not yet, if ever. You tell yourself that if a man truly loved you then it wouldn't matter, because he would love all of you regardless. But deep down inside that sounded like a phrase someone made up who believed it was the journey not the destination when they failed to win a prize. It sat in the back of my mind. Would I ever find someone who would love me enough to handle my ups and downs, my left and right, my ins and outs, my ons and offs? Someone who embraced the raw material that makes up the core of a human being. A core that swings two ways and that will never be one?

I am a woman just like any other. More or less. A woman that sits on the toilet and grabs her stomach fat and curses it more than a wet dream that gets interrupted. A woman that swallowed a lot of dead phone calls that never rang. A woman that sits inside her being wondering why or when the rest of the world was going to get it. When the rest of the insane would understand the sanity of love. Love that bursts from an excited pulse that wakes your heart and has no calm that the world seemed to subscribe to. And live by.

You live like the woman that you are. Not the one you mean to be. The one that grabs that fat and says ok, this is me. I may not like it but I face it. I face the world with an honest grin and show my flaws, my insecurities through human gestures and dialogue that springs out of the mouth before any censure from the brain. That sings when no one else breathes. That doesn't have smooth hair to flip and lets a day go by without a hair dryer. And then there's the passion. The passion that is a blessed bitch.

I have so much passion that it hurts more than the average person so I have to be careful. In my experience, guys could wander in and out of your life as if they never thought about you unless they were standing right in front of you. I was far from standing in front of any of them and thanked God a bit because it would piss me off if Carter tried to walk back into my life. But I knew I would accept him back. The question was, how many times and how much longer was our come and go relationship going to last? Nothing lasts forever, thank God. Right?

Truth is, there is no box for that other girl. "Other" can be anything and being something other than "other" leaves you with nothing.

CHAPTER 32

April 1, 2010 – AXIS II

I opened a case with Axis II today. AXIS II. He did not have any psychotic features, he did not have chronic paranoid schizophrenia or a bipolar condition. Somewhere along the way he developed a learned behavior that was juvenile. He wanted to be taken care of so did his best to continue his mantra.

"The meds aren't working. I'm still hearing voices." That pole he rested on changed when he was told he was going to move to another Ward where the doctor had a tendency to conserve 90% of his patients. The doctor on the Ward he currently inhabited tended not to conserve as much, but that doctor was on vacation, so another doctor was covering his unit. Different doctor, different verdict. To be conserved or not to be conserved: that is the question. And the collective plethora of particles that determined that answer was one thing: a problem. What are the questions we need to ask and where are the answers? It's not black and white like life or death which presents a serious problem. The destiny of a patient had so many elements for or against their locked or unlocked future placement that it continued to daunt, and haunt me, like Hamlet's skull. Axis II could have been discharged to the HIH program, but he refused it. So does that mean his alternative is a locked IMI? Possibly. It depended on so many factors: the doctor you happen to have treating you, the social worker that had his or her input after engaging in good or bad conversations with the patient, the discharge planner and the resources they were or were not available to find in the community that week, the nursing staff with their eyes and ears that may or may not have witnessed incidents on the unit or, if they happened to come across some good or bad behavior from a patient that may or may not be reported in rounds, and could or could not be locked on a page in the medical chart of the patient, and the list went on and on and more on. And that list was only piled up by employees of the county inside the hospital doors. What about the other list: the family, the friends. Would or should or can they take a patient back into their home? How educated were they on the ins and outs of the system. How much did they know about mental health or did they want to? Was there shame that held a fork to a closed mouth that was hungry? The loose elements that determined the fate of a patient were just that, loose. Obviously each case is bruised with lots of lost colors but shouldn't there be a more solid cement way of deciphering the future life of an individual? I didn't have answers and didn't know all the questions to ask but somewhere inside the wobbly line of contemplation, I knew there was a serious problem that had to be addressed. Some how, some way. Simply put: if Axis II wasn't moved to the other ward there is a very fair chance he would have been discharged already. But the doctor on that ward happened to be on out that week so…his life the next year would be a different piece of cake to have and eat it too. So he was moved.

"He's going to be an interesting case." The doctor looked forward to treating him. The social worker informed him of the move and the potential conservatorship and panic mode set in.

"I can't be conserved. I was conserved before."

"Where?" He continued to leave his past a blank page.

"I don't want to talk about that."

"OK, that's your choice, but I am here to help you and if you don't want to be conserved you're going to have to listen to me."

"I'm listening, my medication isn't right."

"OK, well some of the treatment team think you are hospital couch surfing and using this place as a place to keep a roof over your head."

"That's not true. I'm still hearing voices." He burst out of his chair and I knew his fear and frustrations but I didn't understand why he didn't understand he was now in a place where that mantra was going to bite him in his pigeon toed feet.

"Listen, you are going to the other ward. So when you sit down with the doctor, tell him what meds have worked for you."

"Abilify. I told them Abilify but no one is listening to me. I think they want to conserve me because I didn't agree to that program."

"No, that's not it."

"I have a discharge plan. You spoke to my friend. He said I could stay there and he would take me to the clinic to get my meds."

"Then when the doctor sits down with you, you tell him you have a plan. You want to try Abilify and your friend is going to take you in. But you have to stop this bullshit about not wanting to take a bus to your friend's house because you'll jump your head out the window if we don't give you some other form of transportation."

"I'm trying to get a hold of my sister to see if she can help me. But

I only have a dollar worth of quarters left and that phone takes my quarters every time."
"Then use the other free phone." Over and over and over there was a spinning winding whirl of excuses that always left us back at the same place.
"I have a place to go but need my meds straight." He was transferred later that day against his will. I didn't stay around to see the transfer. I am sure it wasn't pretty, just like Belly Dancer's discharge to the bus stop was flooded with screaming at her mother and red swollen pockets of skin beneath her eyes. I'm sure the move entailed some madness. I would have to check in next week and continue to work on the plan. I knew deep down inside he was going to be conserved because he wasn't listening or wasn't getting it, which was beyond frustrating because I didn't think he had a mental illness which meant he was capable of helping himself, I think. At least more than the remaining 90% of the population stuck on the Wards. However, his foggy upbringing made it hard to decipher how his nurturing could have led to behaviors of a person that leaned on a system that adhered to the mentally ill…but didn't for personality disorders. Where are the beds for those patients? I wasn't familiar with Axis II personality disorders and knew it was going to be a massive learning experience. So far I knew one thing: An Axis II was either a chronic manipulator who was playing a sick game, or they were a chronic manipulator unable to play any game because that's all they know. Somewhere along the way they incrementally built a life of victimization from outside experiences. It was not a born condition but a result of the experiences they happened to have in their life. But at this point it seemed too late, because if he didn't realize he was a chronic 'I am a victim' slave to himself then could he be helped? He was a victim of himself. Could an orange find juice again once the sun dries it out over time and turns it into a prune? Oranges don't turn to prunes but they might as well because the deconstruction was going to be that hard.

I walked through the locked door to the Ward ready to call it a week when I rounded the corner and ran into Oreo. Oreo was one of my other upon other open cases that I rarely had time to see because it was quantity not quality, remember? She was originally on another Ward when she called 911 on a Saturday night because she couldn't breathe. She was fat and young and back from St. Luke's Medical Center.

"Hi." She said it flat with some enthusiasm somewhere detected deep inside.

"Oreo, you're back."

"Yeah, I had these chest pains, these horrible chest pains. They said I was going to die if I don't stop smoking."

"Then you need to quit. You don't want to die, do you?"

"No. Well, sometimes." She cracked a tiny smile. So did I. I didn't find it funny, sort of, but we shared a brief moment of understanding. She spoke a truth and as terrible as that truth sounded sometimes the truth is funny.

"He wrote a pretty well put together list." I sat scared that my spelling of communicate would show an outside source helping Wheelchair write a list to change the destiny of his life. When he couldn't spell 'neics' (nieces) and 'nefus' (nephews).

"I think he can go back to his sisters." The social worker worked to confirm this plan and sent a nod to agree with this turning point. He seems to have a plan and cognitive ability to be able to show some sort of life plan.

"Here you have a guy who's been given a hard deck of cards. He needs some guidance. We'll discharge him to his sister."

His guidance rested on having someone stand beside him and come up with some goals. Goals he came up with on his own. I wasn't going to feed him any words to describe his future. He could do that on his own. He just needed someone there to help him spell 'back', (not 'bak'), and write a sentence that stood strong enough to sell the doctor his freedom.

And he wrote his list with the sides of his hands rubbing his dead legs in anxious uncertainty in between those lines he made on his paper, but he wrote them. All 15 of them. On his own. And I could sit there in rounds and hear that he was okay not to be conserved. One stop of, 'can you talk to me for a second?', and a lean against a wall while we worked out his goals that he wrote down in a half pencil that held his freedom gave him some purpose. He could do what he wrote on the paper, because he wrote it by himself.

April 5, 2010 – SMART

I opened a case on Smart today. Smart was a 62-year-old man with schizophrenia.

"I want to talk to my brother. Dr. Ted H. Smith. He's a doctor in Oakland at Berkeley Center. I need to speak with him so he can send me some money."

"When's the last time you spoke with him?"

"Ah…years ago. 15 years ago. He's a surgeon." And he was. His father was a doctor also and no one in the family had dealt with him since his first to fifth mental break. He had been in board and cares and on the street for years.

"I heard you went to Berkeley. What did you graduate in?"

"Political Science." He had old tired eyes shaped like the pupils of a cat. And they were sucked into his head and lost somewhere in his brain.

April 8, 2010 - LAAAADA

Smart left yesterday. So much for that open case. The Stage is leaving tomorrow. There goes another one. I'm back where I started with less than the requirement. And staff meeting is tomorrow so things are awesome.

April 15, 2010 - ECT

I found out in rounds that electric shock therapy could only be administered voluntarily. But, apparently at Central hospital they were doing it all the time.

"They are doing it to teach the residents." Just like I could get a patient to sign a form without them really knowing the nuts and bolts, I am sure over at Central they pitch the program in such a way to get that "voluntary" signature. It's not voluntary if you are psychotic. So the patients were electric minions to train the thirsty residents. Sick.

Later I found out that you are supposed to try five.   FIVE medications before you consider ECT.   And meds take 3-6 months to see if they work.   These patients were being zapped about a couple of med attempts a few weeks into the job.   Sicker.

April 18, 2010 - SCHOOLED

I got schooled today in rounds about Axis II.   The Dinosaur spoke about this existential method used to handle Axis II patients. Instead of going back and forth with me proposing options and him blocking them and me saying well then this and that back in my face then OK well that again, the swirly whirling raging waters could be handled by another approach.

"You agree with the patient."   His calm demeanor and sage like fashion always got my attention.

"If he says the meds aren't working then you agree with him and talk it through."   The Dinosaur went on to explain how Axis II needed confidence and someone to take care of him so the approach had to be from a different, motherly, angle.   I agreed with his method for dealing with Axis II.   But I also felt there was a strong line between a positive supportive approach and coddling.   And I wasn't sure how to approach the difference.

April 20, 2010 – THE SHORELINE PITCH

The Stage is gone.   It was sad.   It hit me later that night after my steam at the gym.   I walked out naked and sat in the quiet room.   No one ever walked naked in the woman's locker room and I wondered if there was some unwritten rule and people were so wowed by my I could give a rats ass and love being naked so get over it and into it attitude that no one dared to say anything.   But I didn't care.   Maybe somehow I could start a trend.   Anyway, I sat down to unload the remaining steam from my skin and next to me was a woman who looked just like The Stage.   She was asleep on a chair with a towel across her head and I thought about The Stage during the interview today for Shoreline.

"I'm going home."   She had actually recently acknowledged that her husband was not the Queen of Spain and exchanged a few phone calls with him. But it was too late.

"Well, The Stage, you can't go home. You have to take steps and the first one is to go to Shoreline."

"What's Shoreline?" The representatives of the naked hell hole that was far from the naked liberties I enjoyed in the woman's locker room was doing her best to sell the place.

"We have a great patio." A cement block with a blue tarp.

"Do you smoke?" Their faces lit up like smoking was a good thing. "We have another great patio just for you to smoke." But no.

"No. I don't smoke." The air was squeezing out of the sails we needed to make this happy transition.

"I go home, I go home to my husband. I have to cook for my children. You understand, you mothers. I'm sorry my English is bad." Her English was fine, just fine. She was an immigrant in a foreign mental country of a brain and she didn't think we understood her.

"The Stage, you are conserved." The Shoreline rep threw out the word to a stone face. It took me weeks to understand the meaning of that word and I wondered if they made it hard on purpose so people wouldn't know what it meant. What about locked up against your will. Everyone understands the truth, don't they?

After the interview Shoreline asked if I would come be their liaison. "I wouldn't be caught dead there." Shock screwed up the eyes of her face and I stood still. What.

The Stage went later that day. I didn't hang around to watch her go. She asked to see me but I said no. It was just one of those days that felt bad and truly sunk in four hours later after a relaxing steam, and a tired old woman that reminded me of The Stage sleeping beside me. She was in the quiet room and would soon go home.

"How are things?" I was at Sampson's, again. And realized again would be again and again tomorrow and next month and next year and probably for the rest of my life. Forever. It was the same old interview with my same old replies. Which I guess I should be grateful for because it meant that my meds were working for quite some time at this point. I guess I should have been happy or relieved or something but it was boring. I was boring.

"Good. Things are good." I nodded my head at the truth.

"How are things at Ocean?
"Eastside. I moved hospitals. It's good. But it's not forever."
And I drove home thinking. What am I doing? Why am I here? I know a truth. The writings real. The stories. The sadness. The story.

CHAPTER 33

JOURNAL ENTRY – I GET IT, THANK GOD - 2010

Why
Why
Why
Did you call me
Or even try to
Be
Back in my life
After all the years
Past.

I cried
I smiled
I loved
You.

Dean called me today. Lets take a moment and hear that one in. Okayyyy..whatt? I was half confused. He left a message saying that he tried to reach me but had the wrong number and had left a few voicemails on some other person's phone. He wondered if I was mad at him since he didn't hear back from me. Ah...more WHAT?!? First there was Ryan, ten years later. Then there was Dean, five years later. What next? Carter?

Where was he going to fall on the rolling hills of events called my life. The undying question mark that never gave any full answer. So I wrote him an email. By this point we hadn't spoken in two years. Two years really isn't a long time when you think about all the on and off years and dead years that snailed by within the decade.

The email I sent him replied back like death on the computer screen. Death.

And what he wrote will never be told.

What I felt at that moment burned through a pen when I wrote a poem about it. It was time to hang my heart on a dirty towel rack and trash it after I used it to clean the cement floors of my loft. Was it the poem that should have been mine? Maybe he doesn't love you. Maybe he didn't enough to say he did. Maybe he did a few fleeting times at some sunken moments when he needed someone. I'm not that maybe someone anymore cause it's not okay. It's time to be me alone in a pulsating heart and mind that can't seem to let go of what? Of pain, ungiving, unwanted, unfair love. Somewhere along the line you think the void of unclarity will find its way to freedom. And thanks to that poem, mine did. I was free from forever of I think so, maybe, sort of, possibly, kinda, more or less…finally I realized the diamond of truth. Alone in the self is not so alone when you break yourself free of that part of the self that holds onto, waits for, prays that somehow someday someone will get it. Be it. Be all those moments you kept to your living dying heart in the hope life will make it what you think you are or should be. It's just fine as it is.

Men. They love me. They leave me. But they come back. Cause they don't forget. But they don't change. People fundamentally don't change. The id is drilled into the core of the being and the rest builds, evolves, and works around it. I knew time allowed me to clean the memories of unrequited love but also knew that welcoming my past back into my life opened a door to re-know my feelings. I pulled out old poetry books and realized that Dean was my first love poem. He was my first passionate pulse between the words of exchange that tantalized my brain and found words on a page. There were pages of heart fierced into the sheets of poetry made heavy by the testosterone of love. Lust. Wanting. Needing.

And I felt so much. I was speared with my own words on the pages of my life. I had so much intense passion that was once felt and not disappeared. That love never disappears when you write it all down. And can look it up and read it. I loved certain people hard for a period in my life in the intense nature of my ways. I read a period of time of fueled crisp fire that stood in its millimeter black ink above the surface of the page and sang heartfull, heartache, heart drowned, heart there alone on a curb by a rocky bedrock. You write and leave out things here and there. You try to write a truth so others can hear and know or feel something honest when you aren't one to make characters or plot lines to make a story or make sense of any of the trunks of magic diamonds and pirate juice of the human chest of love. I think I told the truth across the pencil page. I read poetry from before. Before I lost feelings deep inside my holes. Before I woke up one day and was a little better. Before was before. And I didn't recall that time before cause it bled so hard in the ears and ripped down my spine while flurrying my mind with blank nothingless love that was sprayed on my heart. Every day. Praying that one day it would be before. Before I loved. Before I felt like red gems glistening in a thin lake. And now my past contacts me after peels of onions had been flossed away.

So now what?

Time had healed the wounds of rejection but the writing keeps it alive. And bleeding. Writing has been my best friend my whole life. It is my eternal salvation and has saved me from myself beyond a number of times. It held my hand through dark times, confused states of mind, passionate cries from the heart, and was my only true undying immortal friend. It was the only thing that knew me and let me be myself without any judgments. It was my only release from myself and it captured moments of periods of my life in raw form. But there was a tradeoff. It kept me alive and free but could come back and haunt me when I returned to it. I had to keep it real to the truth of my mind at the time and the plot of my life that surrounded it. You can't ignore what you were like as much as it pains you to read it. The trunk chest of skeletons that sat in my past but were kept alive on the page would never disappear. I guess it's nice to see how aspects of you change through your writing but you can never escape from those writings. You have to face your fire even when it burns.

Reading poems or passages about previous lovers in my life was a stamp of feelings that I could scratch and sniff. Over time the scent fades but the sticker remains. I have loved a few men in my life. And I find a kick, not in the chest thankfully, but somewhere on my side of irony and hilariousness to see them return. But it's too hard for some people. For the men that I've loved. They sprinkled my life enough to make a stain. They did their best to balance my passion with what they know. Which is like trying to live inside a world that has no bullshit, no lies, no female craft of sexy syrupy breasts falling across the chest.

The woman that does as she wants will never be edible.

Love in life is pretty simple in its wild complexities. Even if your psychotic or schizophrenic or depressed or turning your heart out to the outsider world when it's smashed inside your freedom. You have your instinct. Your inside mind, heart, soul, passion to scream its truth to your conscience self. After all the deadfull nights of lostness you have one certainty. Your truth sits happily inside your heart. Philosopher kings have always spoken of the evolving nature of truth and the human condition that attempts to define it, seek it out and make it known. Living a life fueled by a desperate desire to find truth is like chasing a Godlike spirit that is always ahead of you somewhere in the evolving nature of life and the realities of the human condition. But I know one truth that I can say without any hesitation. I love my family. I love my friends. I love the people that are my own. Those that are there for me down and out and in-between and hard or soft or yes or no. They are the force that keep me alive and make me be. And my being would always be rooted in an undying need to seek out truth. No matter what.

My agonizing pursuit of truth had always seemed to get me in trouble. In relationships, in jobs, in my existence in society. We don't live in a world that champions truth all that much. We are perpetually sucked into adhering to societal demands to fit in. And when you fight that gravity that constantly tries to pull you into a black hole of bullshit you will always walk a different line.

CIVILIZED ACCOMMODATIONS

Change is nurture working at its hardest.

Nature is your mind that you can never escape.

When nurture hits your mind

You try to tame the beast

Of the nature of your being

When really after all the runs, walks, hikes, yoga, wheat grass injections

You'll still be the nature of your beast.

The person you were drilled into the planet

By you

Since the break into the world

Of living life.

Nature versus nurture

Has so many threads of debates when really

It is simple:

Nature is your being

Nurture is what happens to accommodate it.

When you accommodate your nature

You die a little

Inside

But maybe it's better for the rest of

Civilized civilization.

Or is it?

JOURNAL ENTRY – THE VOID - 2010

I have finally become accustomed to being alone. Thank God. I don't search for someone else to hold my hand or rest beside me in my bed. I have finally become that person that I never thought was possible. Self-full. A self. I don't know if it was the meds or sheer time alone. Did my former untreated manic depression breed profound loneliness and now with medication my brain stopped screaming for help, for someone or something other than itself? I was relieved that I finally did not suffer loneliness. I had actually managed to become that person I longed to be ten years ago. A person that wasn't eaten alive by herself. A person that wasn't obsessed with finding a man to fill the void. I was finally free from the words I treaded water in while I wrote one time on my fire escape and wondered if my naked masturbator would ever return.

THE VOID

I feel it deep inside.
Give me more.
Feed me.
Run for me.
It speaks.
And nothing else matters.
I can't hear my body, nor do I listen to my mind.
The voice is an empty hallow place that needs something that you can't seem to place.
Frozen yogurt?
Love?
It seems to like being fed stuff that numbs the body and mind.
I can do that.
Anything to make it happy.
It knows how to make me feel good.
I give it everything it wants.
Without knowing it will only grow.
And eat me alive.
I am lonely and the voice is the only thing I hear.
My only sad friend.
But it's all I have.
As I lose myself.
The voice becomes you.
And you listened to it to avoid feeling alone.
And you do everything it says.
Feeding it to make it shut up.
You want to starve it.
But you can't.
And the loneliness grows.
Your life becomes a slave to the voice.
Then you realize that voice is the void.
The lonely spirit that runs through humanity and engulfs innocent lovers of life.
You have to fight your ass off to kill the beast.
That never really dies.
You grew it while being alone.
You thought it was your only friend.
Forgetting the difference between good and bad friends.
Or having no friends at all.

Loneliness and hypomanic depression.

JOURNAL ENTRY – YES, I DID IT, WHY…I'M NOT SURE

I lowered my Lamictal. It was the first time in my life since my first mental throw down on my brain that I actually did such a thing. I started biting off bits and pieces of a whole mind slowing nugget and things did change. I didn't sleep for an entire night but float slept simmered along the surface of my stale sheets. My veeg started opening up like a night blooming jasmine pretty much all day like it does after a woman jumps at the seams of an internal high following a releasing climax. I wasn't thinking that much about sex but my body sure was, as it was charged to the point that hypersexuality was finally my middle name again. There were also a few incidents at work beside the usual skipping words in my notes or running through emails like a speed demon with fire on my fingertips. I used the wrong key for an unlocked door a couple times in a mental rush to go somewhere in front of some co-workers who were totally perplexed. Some people said I looked different because I was up and peachy high. Happy. An animated tree. But I also found once again those irritable moments that jumped just beneath my skin to boil the blood that rested against the walls of my flesh. Yes, my eyeballs started to burn from skipping days of sleep and anxiousness fired my heels that tried to keep up with my legs spinning down the street, but it didn't make me want to slow down. Then the pain and frustration of life on a stick of borderline hell set back into the almighty center of my brain. Time became a nightmare again as the clock struck down on my head never and I waited for someone to stop in and talk some sense into me.

"Doctor Loberg." Scribble scribble.
"Yeah, I bite too little off too much and my neck started to burn when I sprayed Chanel on my freks." I started to get that rash that people get if they don't ease into Lamictal and the tiny bumps sitting on my collar bone were slightly alarming and a swap onto my chest that I did too much pulling back."
"Did anything change in your behavior?"
"I had a serious falling out with the light bulb."

"Was this around the time you started lowering your meds?"
"I don't know, yes, maybe, no. I don't know." Why is seeking justice considered a manic behavior? Or maybe it built the confidence I needed to turn that light off. The light bulb put me over the edge, not my condition. Yes, my yearning wet slurpee wanted sex and yes, I wasn't sleeping as much but those were physical responses. Behavior surrounding a hypomanic behavior is another thing. I had to get out from under her bulb so went to her supervisor who told me I needed a doctor's note to get away. She made it sound like it was no big deal and the next thing I know I am at some random sick clinic with local fat and cast bearing soldiers, needing a mental evaluation to get the paperwork to switch off her beam. Things snowballed down my sleepless back when I had to see a county psychiatrist who had to make an assessment to get me out of this mess. Bullshit to flag my county file so I could be switched to another supervisor. It was all protocol but that crap that sat in a packet of mental workers' compensation papers turned into the county looking into the claim because it is not a burn from coffee or old toilet paper in the office bathroom shoved up the ass to build a sore. No. Mental distress does not count because you can't see it. Once again we are back where we started and the non-joke of the whole thing is I'm working in mental health to begin with. So once the insurance person came out to ask me questions about my situation living in the light section of Home Depot I was in so deep I couldn't turn around because the cement had already ended the wet zone. Then the program head directed me to human resources who told me they would reassign me to another supervisor. In another county job? Another item as they called it, like we were a line in all the paperwork that the county charred when it ended up in some tree graves? Fuckkkk you and fuckkk that. I dropped the claim and was back with the bulb. But I got to stay at Eastside until the next real thing let me take my heart. And it will. My writing will save me like it always would. In all the shit bearing jobs I've endured it always sailed me through any damnation. It was the salvation through my tormented heat. My shitty jobs, my relentless disappointments in the tires around me, in men, love, society, in fighting the beat of political correctness or letting the beast of truth set steady in the bones of the living.

I would always speak my truth, myself unleashed within an unleashed mind.

Erica Loberg

CHAPTER 34

JOURNAL ENTRY – TASMANIAN DEVIL

I am surprised I am alive. God must have a special department for people who trek through life like the Tasmanian devil. You can read books and memoirs on the bipolar experience; however, most of them I've found to be written by MD's that give their saga through the lens of knowing what bipolar means and how it manifests itself through their academic experience. But what if you live it, and write during it, and have no idea what "it" is?

It's like a scream in your head. All the time. It's persistent, and the body does its best to relieve it. The tongue tries to keep up with rapid thoughts through fast speech, and your legs bolt as they walk hard through the streets and try to appease the frantic pulses of the brain. When it's quiet, it also takes hold of the body, and makes your eyes burn because the body is exhausted and it can't sleep. It's all the same living thing, just sometimes you swing from the chandeliers, and other times you could give a shit about your place in this world, or wear sweats for a living. And all the time, it's a stem in your brain that is rooted in the core. The constant pulse is worse than the highs, or lows. It is your brain, and you don't know any better, because you've had it since you were born. Dramatic, emotional, daring, sensitive, passionate, wild, tired.

Somewhere along the unsteady line of life you learn something to help you know more about yourself. And for me, it was time. It wasn't until years later that I understood my relationship with time. When you are hypomanic all the time your mind runs while the rest of the world lives in normal time. I remember the day before the first day I took my meds. I sat down to write a poem. I didn't want to forget what that terrible world was like. I didn't want to forget the clock I lived in for the last 28 years. I wanted to be grateful for help. I wanted to be happy I took medication and not be one of those manic people who enjoyed the rush. That thought that without their mind racing they couldn't produce good work. You could be creative and take your meds at the same time. Would your writing ever be the exact same? Probably not. But it was a trade off. Do you want to live on fast forward all the time in your VCR mind?

TIME AND THE VCR

Tired but awake
Aware but delusional
Freight trains
Of thought
Burst
From the brain.

Then it becomes silent.
What did I do?
Where did I go?
I have no idea
Because the madness lives in
Mania
Madness that I believe
Earns truth.

And it does
Somewhere
But it's not a job
It's not productivity
It's simply a moment in space
Of severe
Thought brought forth through
Heightened energy
And it's awesome
And quick salvation
From the world
But it doesn't live in the day-to-day mind
I will never have a day-to-day mind
Because time is a nightmare.

Am I going to sleep tonight
And wake up exhausted
Fueled by anxiety
To go where

To do what?
It's an unreal clock telling me the external world is slow and boring
My mind is fast forward all the time
Or on pause
While the world walks in slow motion
And I'm felt alone
Inside.

CHAPTER 35

FINAL JOURNAL ENTRY – I THINK THEREFORE I REMAIN INSANE

I think therefore I remain insane. I have gone through treatment and am finally starting to understand the depths of my existence. I would not change the chemistry of my brain and accept that being bipolar II is being me. And being your authentic self is a great thing. I hope I have shared something for a person out there who is walking around without help or guidance. And that I've opened a creaky door to the truth behind the mentally ill and our treatment of those sick inside their brain in a white-roomed wall. We run to a person that slips on wet pavement and help them to their toes, or call 911 when a dog gets hit by a car, but we look the other way, uncomfortable, when someone walks down the street disheveled yelling to nothing in the air. We call 911 after the blood visibly runs down the wrists after a razor blade lunch.

And as I continue down the road of perpetual psychiatric recovery, I realize that I don't know where I am going. That's the tricky thing about mental illness. There is no future. There is only you and the now. How you are now, and how you can be better tomorrow and make that future better than the times you were lying flat on the floor, crying in the shower, staring straight into thin air, or running naked in the streets then kissing a tree while jumping into a ocean that may or may not be water, or exciting yourself into a person or place or thing, then drilling yourself into the ground. This is mental illness, and this is my story.

You will always be inside your insane.